StyleItaliano

Yearbook

2022

Editor: Paola Sammaritano, Edra S.p.A.
Paper, Printing and Binding Manager: Paolo Ficicchia, Edra S.p.A.
Cover: Emanuela Contieri, Edra S.p.A.
Layout: Giorgio Gandolfo, Italy
Typesetting: Barbara Rastelli, Italy

This edition first published 2023

ISBN: 978-1-957260-44-0
eISBN: 978-1-957260-66-2

edra
PUBLISHING

Edra Publishing US LLC
3309 Northlake Boulevard,
Suite 203,
Palm Beach Gardens,
FL, 33403
EIN: 844113980

info@edrapublishing.com
www.edrapublishing.com

Printed by "Rotomail Italia" S.p.A., Vignate, Milan, in March 2023

edra
PUBLISHING

StyleItaliano

Yearbook

2022

STYLE ITALIANO Certified
SHADE GUIDES

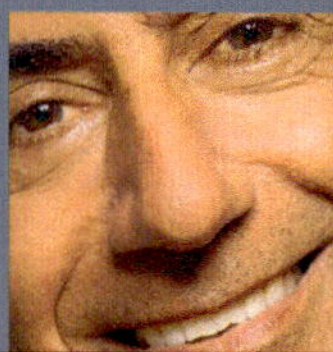

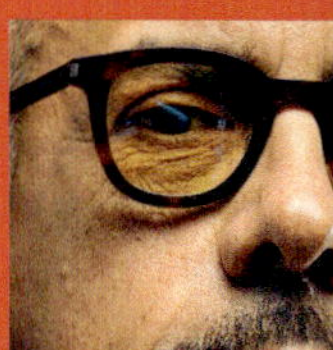

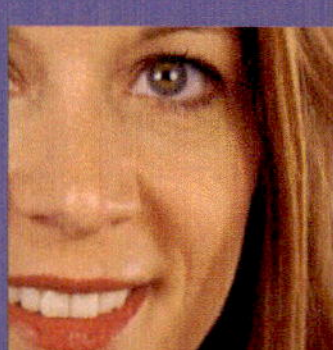

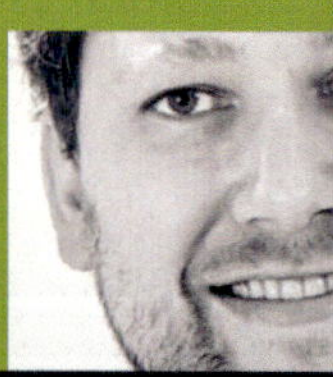

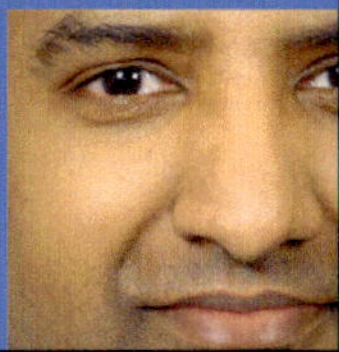

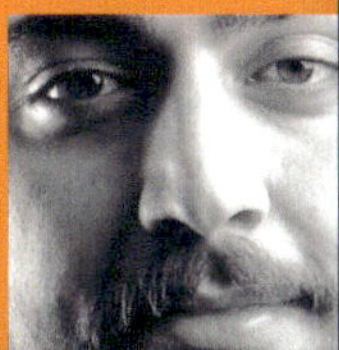

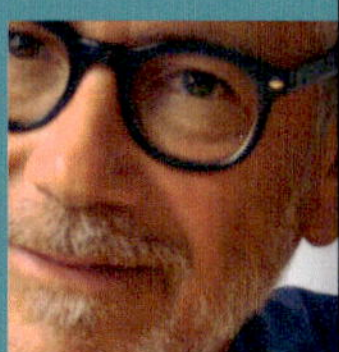

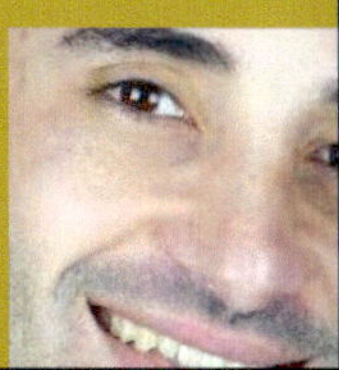

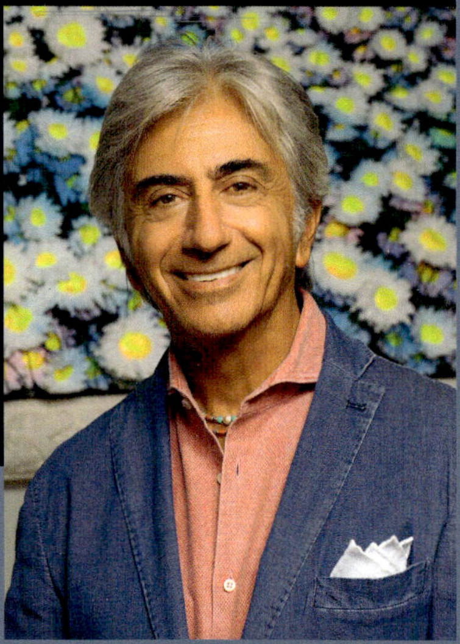

PROF. ANGELO PUTIGNANO MD, DDS

Italy

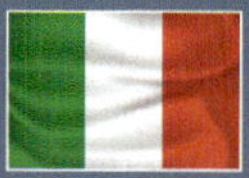

Prof. Angelo Putignano graduated from Medicine Faculty of University of Marche Polytechnic and post-graduated from Dental School of the same University. Since the beginning of his carrier, he lectured internationally on the topics of adhesive and aesthetic restorations.

He became Full Professor in Restorative Dentistry at the Dental Faculty of University of Marche Polytechnic and he is the head of Operative Dentistry and Endodontics Department of the same University.

He also collaborated with the University of Barcelona and University of Marseille as visiting Professor. He also received the Certificate of Excellence as a teacher and dental educator, Tufts University (Boston).

He authored numerous clinical and research articles on aesthetics and adhesive dentistry and is an internationally renowned lecturer on these topics, publishing more than 200 papers.

Lately, he became the Dean of the Dental School of University of Marche Polytechnic.

Over the years, he was active in important dental societies: past President of the Italian Society of Operative Dentistry (SIDOC), Founding Member of the Italian Academy of Esthetic Dentistry (IAED) and Active Member European Academy of Esthetic Dentistry (EAED).

He is co-author of the books *Adhesive Dentistry: the Key to success* edited by Quintessence International (2007), *Indirect Conservative Restoration of Posterior teeth* (UTET 2008), *Layers 2* edited by Quintessence International (2022).

In addition, he is the co-founder of the dental group StyleItaliano which has more than 260000 followers worldwide and proposes precise ideas that help dentists face their own daily challenges in their dental office.

PREFACE

When, 12 years ago, Walter and I started thinking of being able to somehow help the dentist in the choice of material and in its use through repeatable and predictable techniques, while respecting the individuality and abilities of single practitioners, we never thought we would reach so many dentists around the world.
Today, one dentist out of four knows us and knows what we and the group formed around us and to which we owe so much have done in these years.
Simplification and predictability have been the leitmotifs behind our work and focusing on those themes has allowed us to develop techniques and tools to optimize the use of new materials that are transforming aesthetic restoration into one of the most appreciated and requested disciplines in Dentistry.
Our members have followed us on a long and difficult path from their great initial distrust to awareness and competence.
We have shown the highest possible quality dentistry in every country and our members, spread across all continents, are witnesses and interpreters of this.
Many universities have had the opportunity to appreciate how easy our techniques are to teach and how high the students' approval for this is.
And here is our StyleItaliano yearbook where we want to highlight the best interpreters of this dentistry so that everyone can see, know, and understand the philosophy that

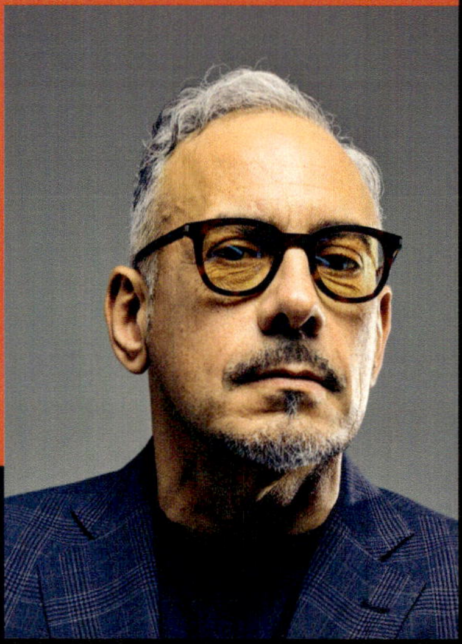

WALTER DEVOTO

Italy

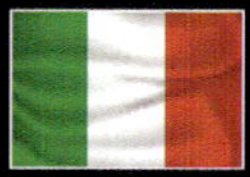

Born in Chiavari the 29/03/1965; graduated with honours in Dentistry and Dental Prothesis in 1991 at the University of Genoa. Dr Devoto has worked as a teacher and demonstrator at the University of Genoa in the undergraduate courses of Dentistry and Dental Prosthesis, teaching Paediatric Dentistry.
From 2000–2004 he taught Reconstructive Dentistry in a course of Laser refinement at the same university. From 2005–2006 he was lecturer at the University of Madrid, Master of Aesthetic Dentistry and from 2005–2009 at the University of studies in Siena, course of Aesthetics and Restorative Dentistry, professorship of Conservative Dentistry. At the moment, he is Lecturer at the International University of Catalonia, Barcelona, for the postgraduate course in Aesthetic Dentistry.
Dr Devoto has been a visiting professor at the Universitè de la Mediterranee (Marseille) in the course of Refinement of Aesthetic Reconstructive Dentistry and was an Adjunct Professor in the University of Marche Polytechnic, Ancona.
Dr Devoto is particularly interested in the field of Conservative Aesthetic Restoration and is the author and co-author of fifty-three articles in specialised international journals.
As a speaker, he has participated in courses and conferences on the subject, both at a national and international level, as well as being a speaker, collaborator, and demonstrator at most of the major European universities. In addition, Dr Devoto is the author of one of the chapters of *Le Guide Estetique* by A Faucher and JC Paris (QDT 2003, France), *Odontoiatria Restaurativa*, by A.I.C. (Elsevier 2009, Italy), *Traumatologia Oral* by A Mendoza (Ergon 2013, Spain), *Endoprotetyka* by M Zarow (Quintessence 2013, Poland), *Licowki* by M Zarow (Quintessence 2020, Poland), and co-author of *Layer 1* and *Layer 2* by J Manauta & A Salat (QDT 2011, 2022).
Since 1996, Dr Devoto has been a member of the Academy of Operative Dentistry. He has also been of the Italian Academy of Conservative and Restorative Dentistry since 1998 and an active member of the European Academy of Aesthetic Dentistry since 2002. Founder member of the Italian Academy of Aesthetic Dentistry. Founder member of StyleItaliano.
As well as running his own private surgery in Sestri Levante (GE) and Portofino (GE), Dr Devoto collaborates with prestigious surgeries throughout Europe, specialising in Aesthetic Dentistry.

PASTE FLASK TECNIQUE: A FRESH CHAIRSIDE STYLEITALIANO FRONTIER IN MODERN DENTISTRY

Restoring anterior teeth in a single session by exploiting quality modern composite is what every dentist would wish for. Patient outcomes and satisfaction are significantly enhanced with a fast, inexpensive solution that does not require special artistic skills and uses a forgiving material with the looks of a ceramic restoration.

All that is now possible thanks to a few techniques for using these new composites, and to the simplification of clinical techniques developed and spread by StyleItaliano. One dentin shade and one enamel are enough to obtain a natural effect. Yet, skills and an artistic sensibillity are needed to obtain a good result. This article proposes an innovative technique that exploits the design which can be achieved in the lab and shows how this technique offers the clinician a series of tools that can significantly simplify on-patient work. This is truly a technique for all that is designed to serve and astonish our patients.

DISCUSSION AND CLINICAL CASE

An eighteen-year-old patient presented complaining about the restorations he had previously undergone by another clinic and that weren't esthetically or biologically appropriate anymore.
The story of this young patient is a story of teeth altered in shape since he was born, with conoid-shaped 12, 22, and 11 (📷 1, 2, 3, 4).

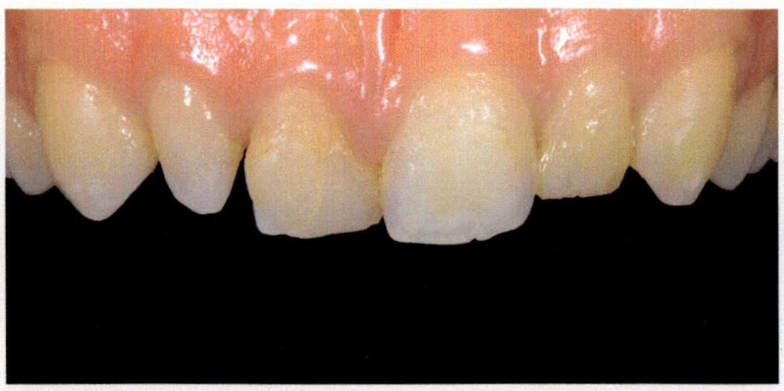

Figure 1 Initial situation. Note the different dimensions of the anterior teeth and the altered gingival contours.

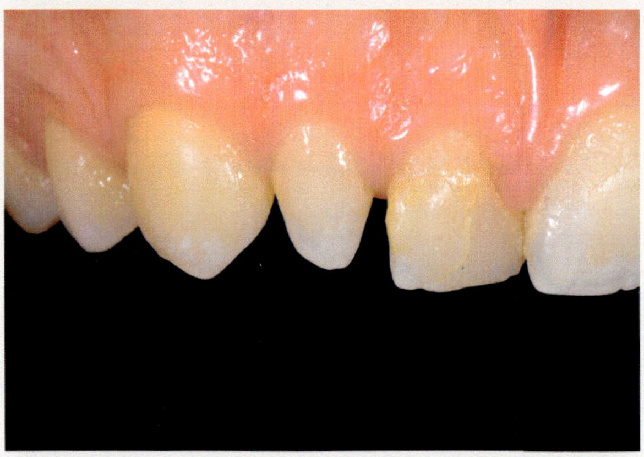

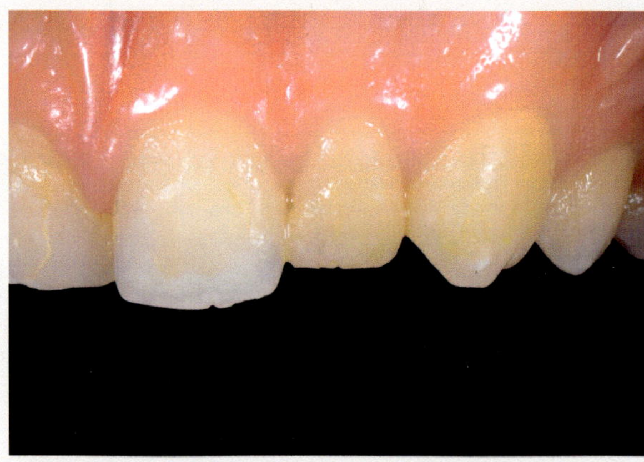

Figures 2-3 Details of the first and second quadrants, highlighting the failure of the previous restoration attempt.

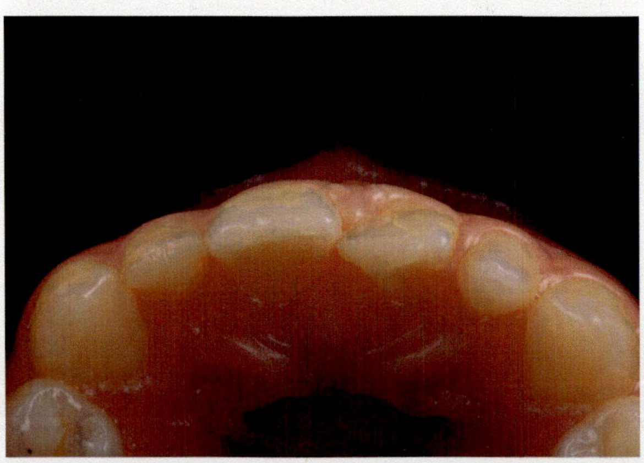

Figure 4 The occlusal view of the anterior group is the most important to set up an additive treatment plan, following the profiles of the two canines.

His previous dentist has added composite material, trying to adapt spaces as best as he could, luckily not preparing the natural teeth and keeping all the enamel intact. We proposed to take an impression and to study his case, with the goal of creating properly shaped additive restorations while aligning them as correctly as possible[1]. In the lab, with the collaboration of our dental technician (Mr. Daniele Rondoni), we could create a new design from the impressions (📷 5, 6, 7) and also create a transparent silicone index to try the result with a mock-up (📷 8).

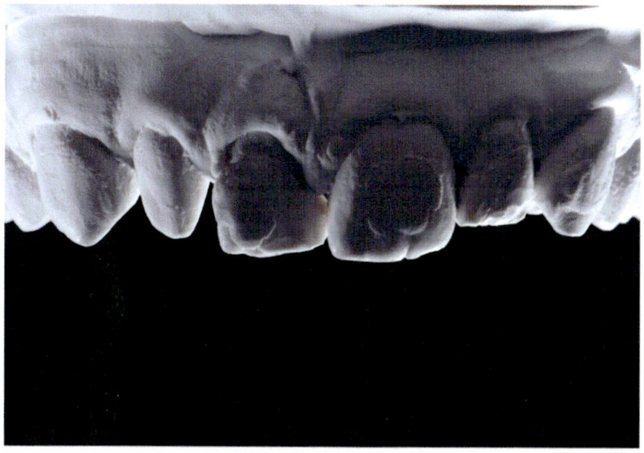

Figure 5 The original model.

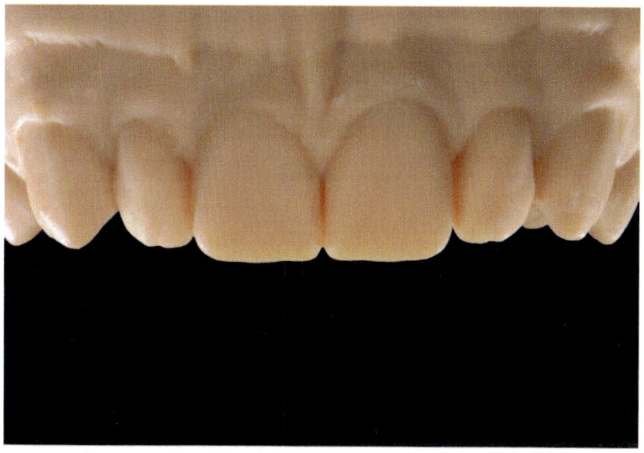

Figure 6 The 3D-printed project.

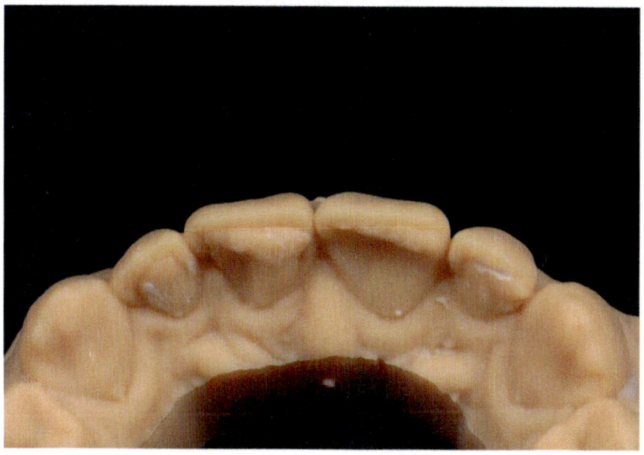

Figure 7 The occlusal view shows the value of the lab project. It would be impossible to plan such case directly chairside.

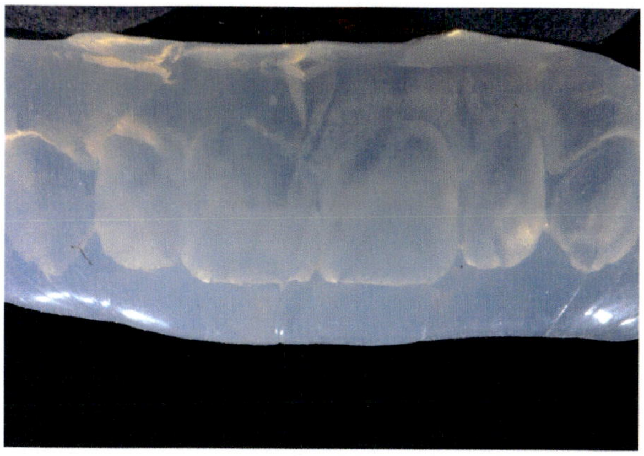

Figure 8 The transparent silicone key realized from the final project, that will guide the mock up.

During the following session, the reaction to the mock-up made us, and the patient, enthused (9, 10). Our modeling showed good esthetics, completely additive, with an excellent space closure between the teeth, which was not simple, even with advanced direct techniques[3].
Moreover, gingival contours seemed optimal[4], thus allowing the whole smile a natural aspect. So, indirect composite restorations (veneers) were proposed to the patient, trusting the long-standing experience with the quality and longevity of these techniques[5].
Limited financial resources did not allow our patient to accept this proposal, hence the idea of an alternative solution. As we already had the new smile designed, and the silicone from the mock-up, why not to directly stamp composite onto healthy teeth?
So we removed the old restorations right away (STYLE DIRETTO bur kit by StyleItaliano, Intensiv Co.) and we modified the gingival contour with a diode laser (Gemini, Ultradent Co.) to improve alignment (11). Then we waited a couple days to achieve perfect healing (12).

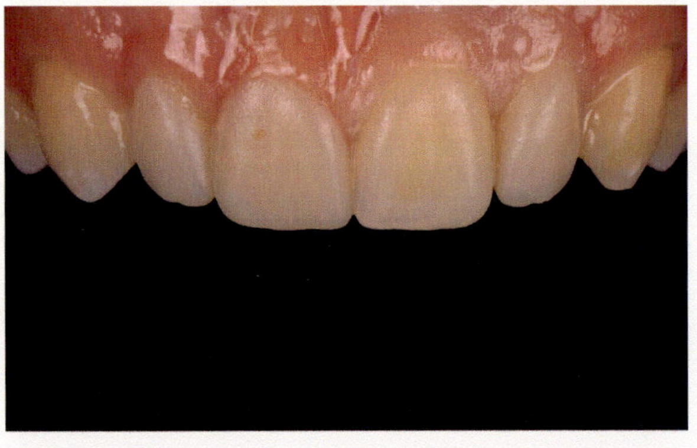

Figure 9 The stamped mock-up, before any gingival modification.

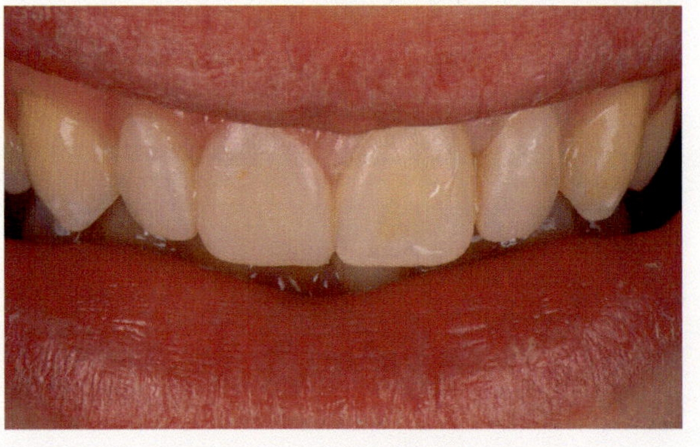

Figure 10 The patient's smile shows naturalness and balance.

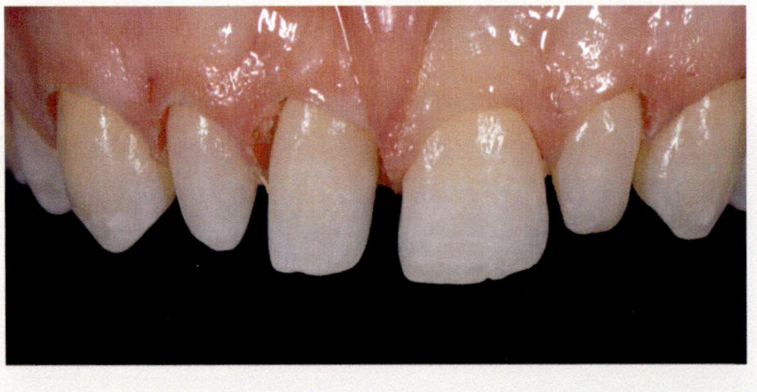

Figure 11 Removal of the old restorations (bur kit STYLE DIRETTO by StyleItaliano, Intensiv Co.) and gingival contour laser modification (Gemini diode laser, Ultradent) to allow, in most cases, immediate restoration.

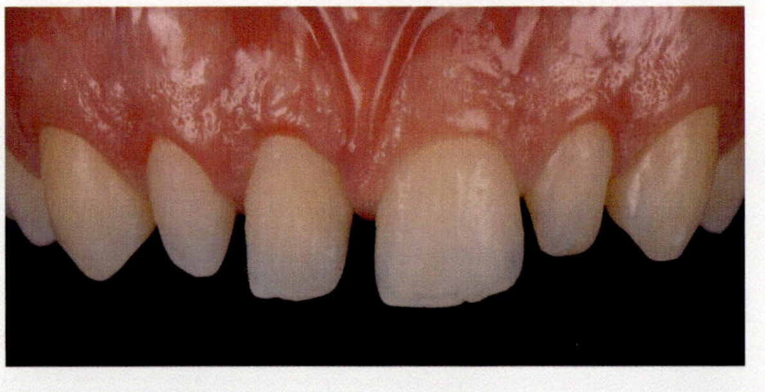

Figure 12 In this case, we waited one week before proceeding to the final restoration, but this choice is optional.

On the following session (about 2 hours) we proceeded tooth by tooth as follows:
A small quantity of enamel composite (Composite Enamel, Optident Co.) was inserted into the silicone key with a suitable instrument (Modella, LM Arte by StyleItaliano) towards the incisal part (13) and, before curing, a body shade was placed to complete the tooth shape (Composite SI1, Optident Co.) (14). Homogeneity was checked through the transparent silicone (15).
Exerting a slight pressure, the silicone key was then placed on the chosen tooth, which had been cleaned but not adhesively treated yet (16). Once position was set, the composite was light cured through the silicone key (CuringPen, Eighteeth) (17).

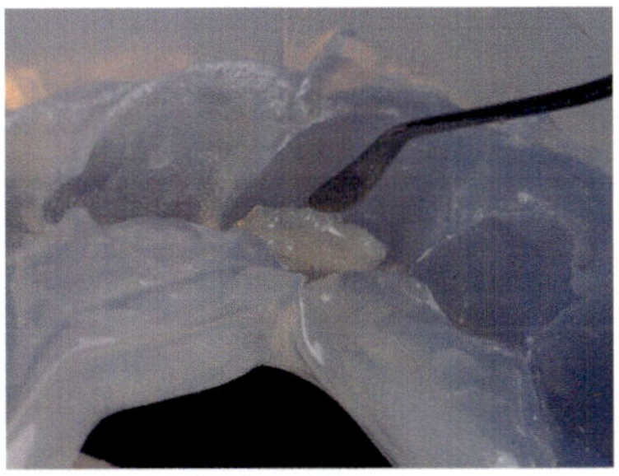

Figure 13 A small quantity of enamel composite (Composite Enamel, Optident Co.) was inserted into the silicone key with a suitable instrument (LM-Arte Modella, by StyleItaliano) towards the incisal part leaving it uncured.

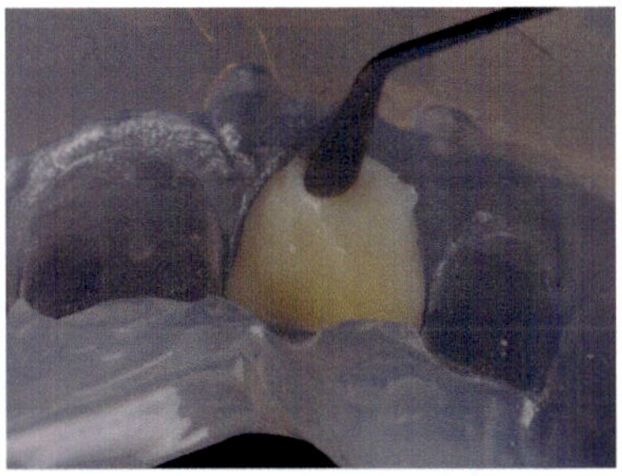

Figure 14 The dentin shade was added (Composite SI1, Optident Co., Henry Shein) on the same tooth.

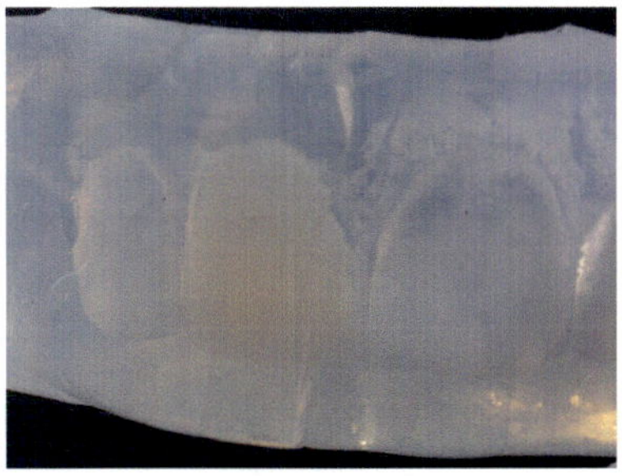

Figure 15 Buccal check for bubbles and defects.

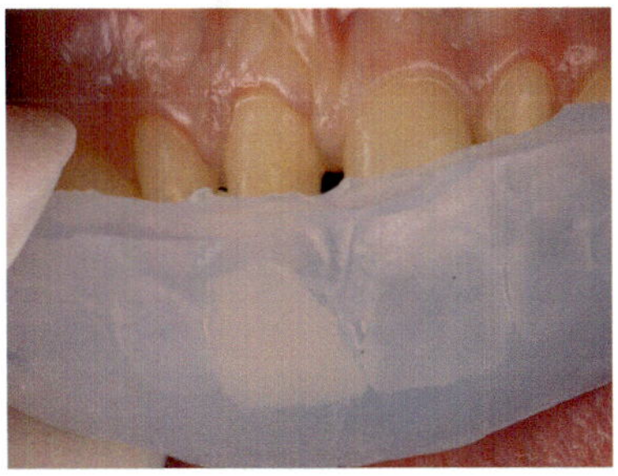

Figure 16 Placement of the silicone key on the untreated tooth.

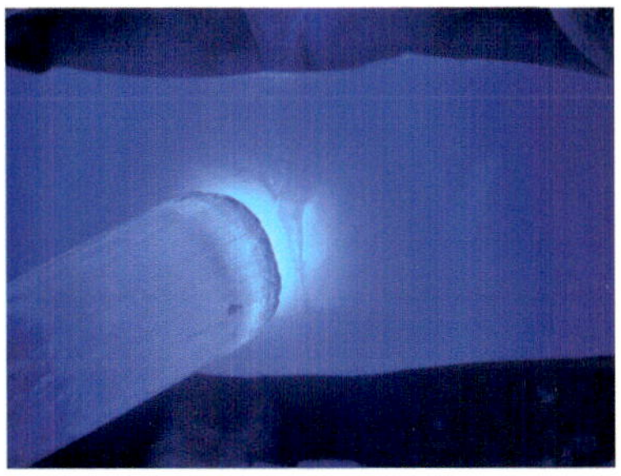

Figure 17 Light curing of the composite through the silicone key (CuringPen, Eighteeth).

Once the key was removed, the veneer sort of magically appeared laid onto the tooth, but unbonded (📷 18). With an appropriate instrument (kit LM-Arte Fissura by StyleItaliano) the veneer was delicately removed (📷 19) and finished outside the mouth (burs kit STYLE FINALE by StyleItaliano, Intensiv Co.).
The result was exciting. The random mix of the two shades turned out to be very natural in opacity and translucency (📷 20) thus simulating manual layering[6], which is not easy to obtain for less experienced dentists.

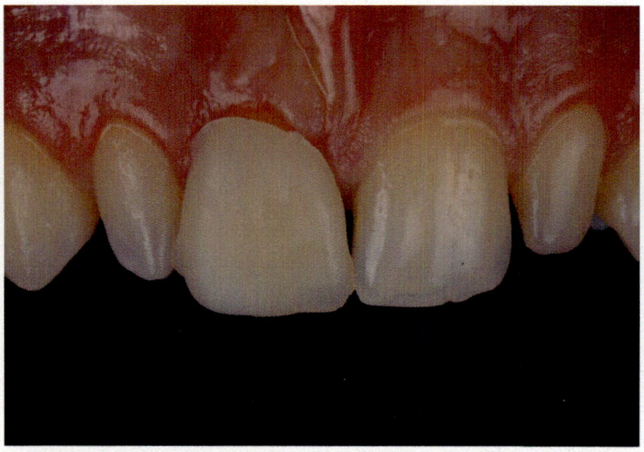

Figure 18 Removal of the silicone key.

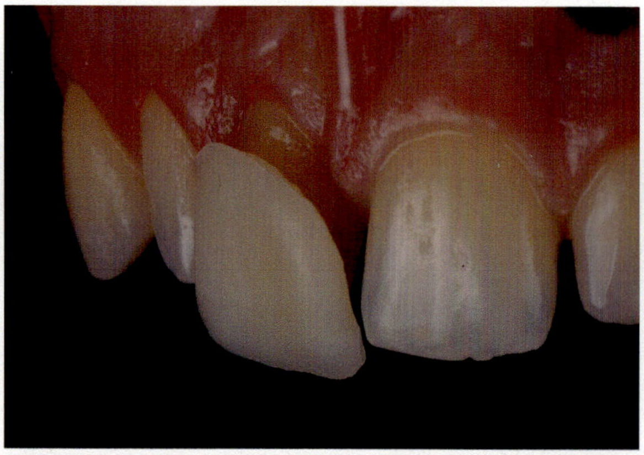

Figure 19 Delicate removal of the veneer with a dedicated instrument (kit LM-Arte Fissura by StyleItaliano).

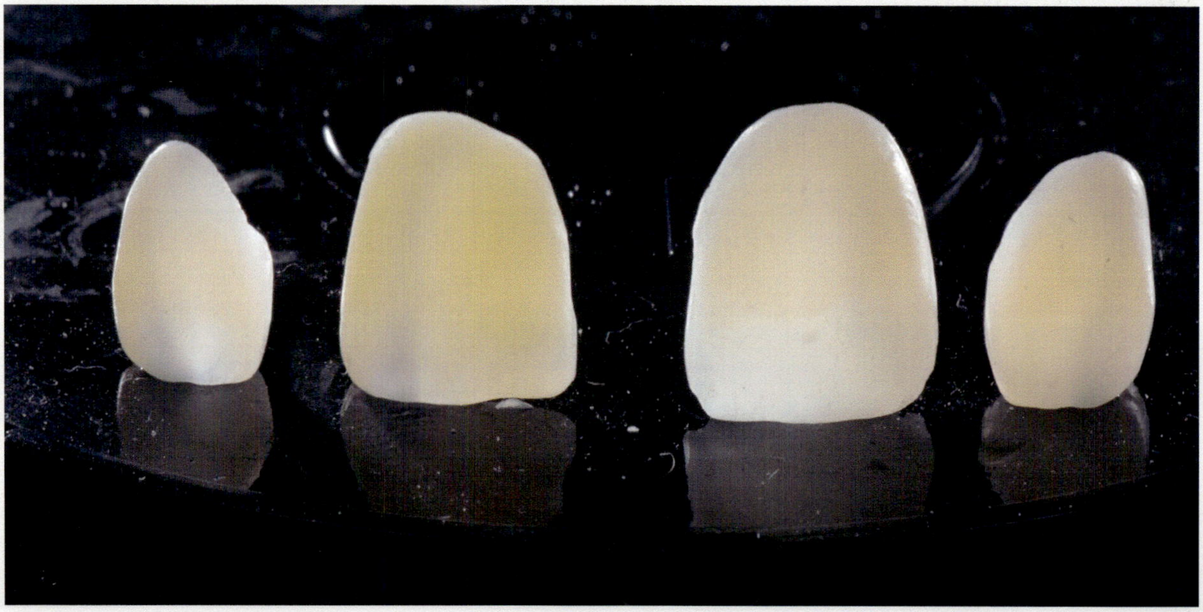

Figure 20 Protocol is repeated on each tooth one by one. Note the good color blend of the enamel and dentin shades.

Repeating the same procedure for each tooth, it is possible to isolate each tooth with the rubber dam and to cement the veneers[7] following the steps we all know: sandblasting (air flow AquaCare), orthophosphoric acid etching, adhesive application, veneer fitting and cementation **(21, 22, 23, 24, 25)**[8].
At the end of the adhesive procedures, it's possible to finish the polishing of the veneers using a dedicated paste (LUCIDA, StyleItaliano) and following the steps to maintain ideal shape and texture[9].

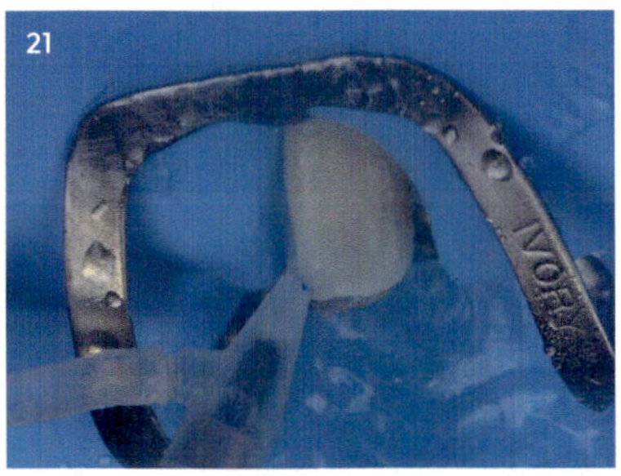

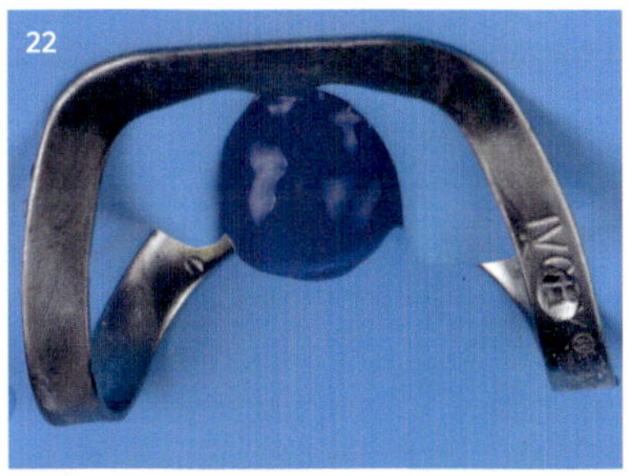

Figure 21 After placing the rubber dam on each tooth, the surface is sandblasted (AquaCare).

Figure 22 Orthophosphoric acid etching (3M).

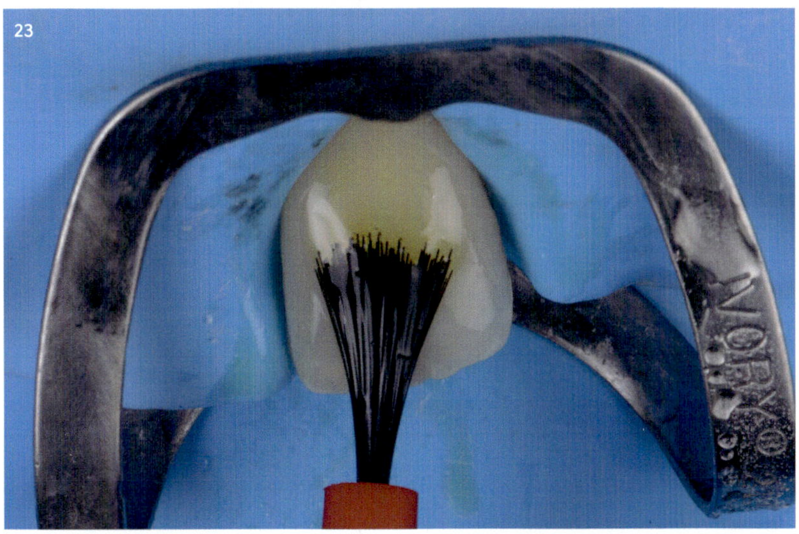

Figure 23 Bonding application (ScotchBond Universal Plus, 3M).

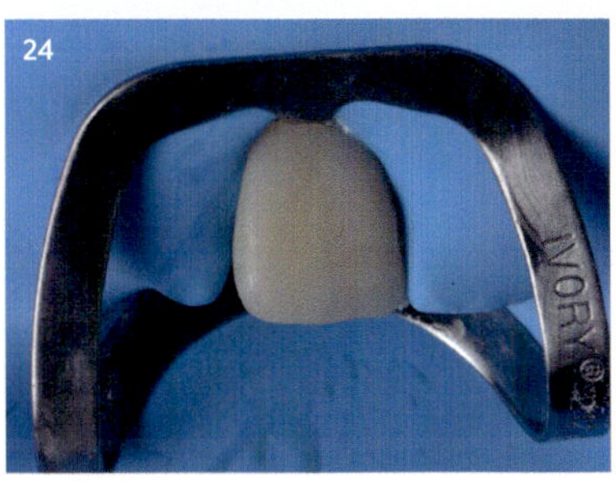

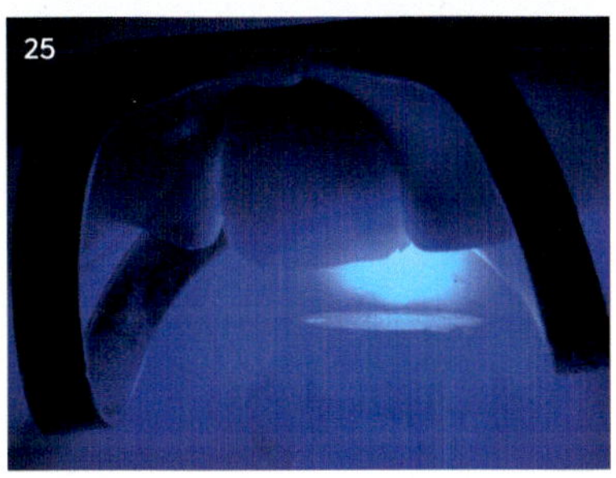

Figure 24 Cementing the veneer with a flowable composite (Composite Multiplo, Optident, Henry Schein).

Figure 25 Final curing.

The final result is very good, considering the simplicity of the proposed solution. Shape and color are naturally integrated[10], in a limited chairtime, without having reduced sound dental structure, and the restoration is possibly repairable and modifiable at any time and with limited expenditure, both for the dentist and the patient (26, 27, 28a, b).

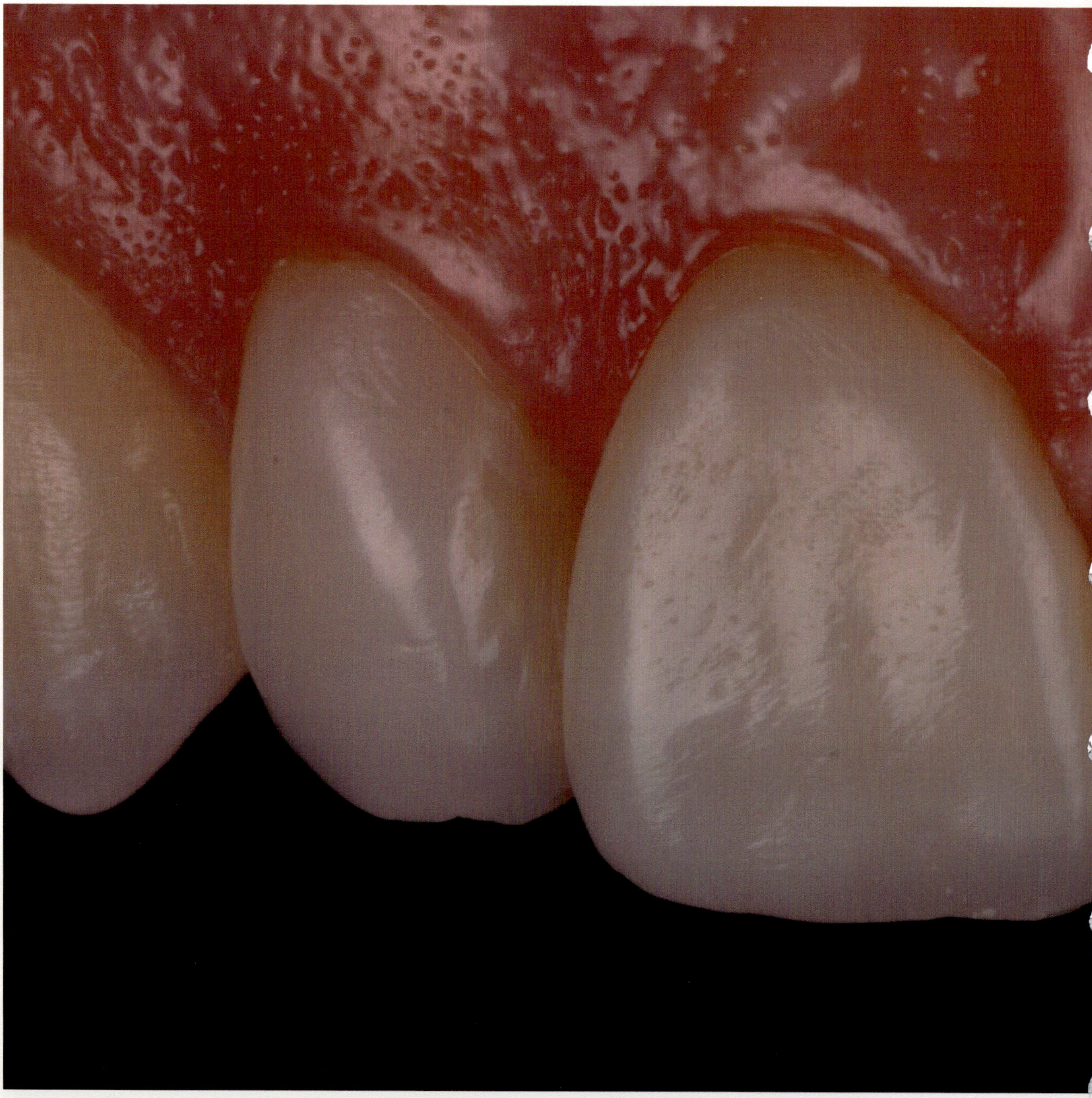

Figure 26 Final result after polishing (Lucida Paste, StyleItaliano).

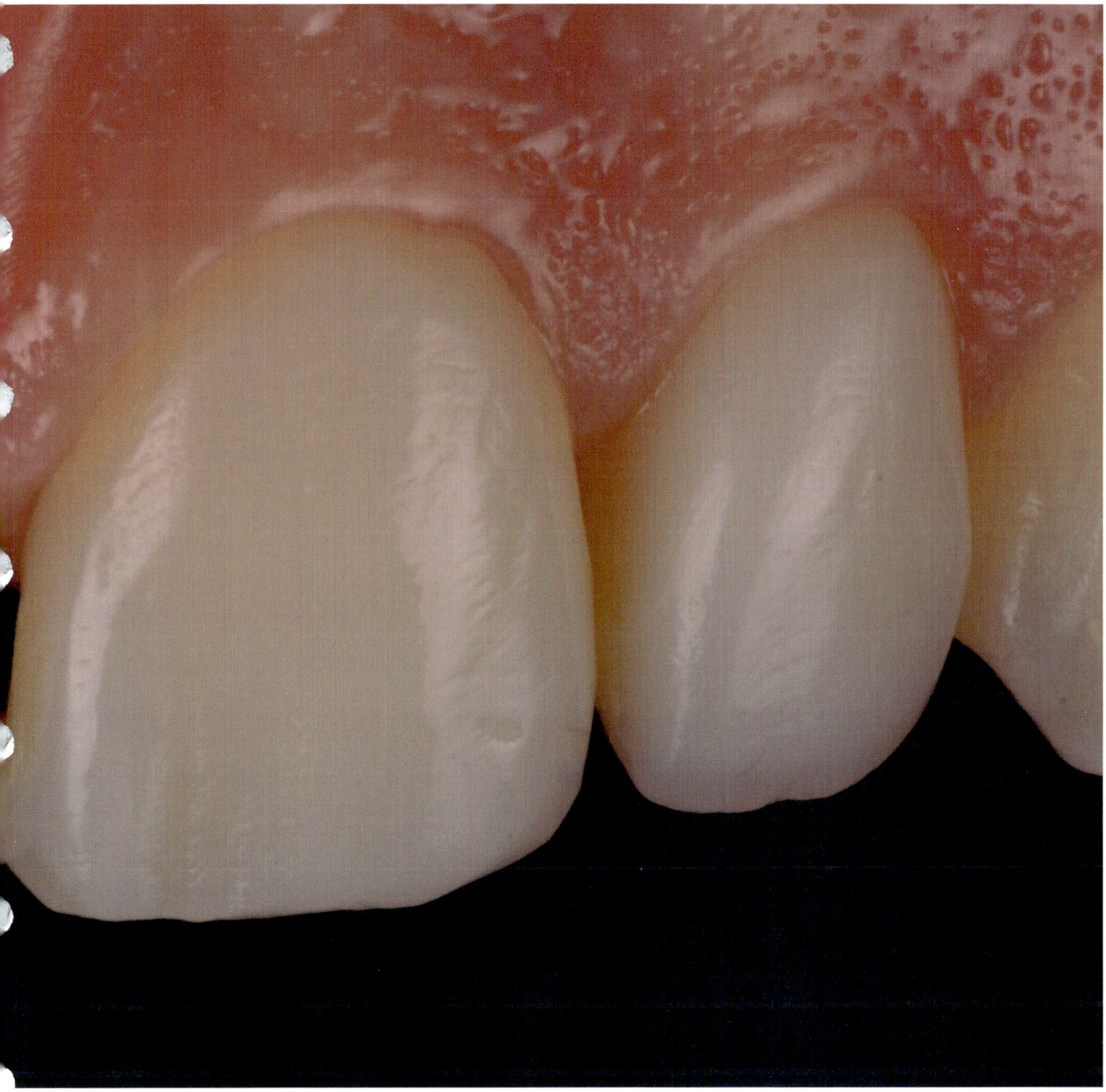

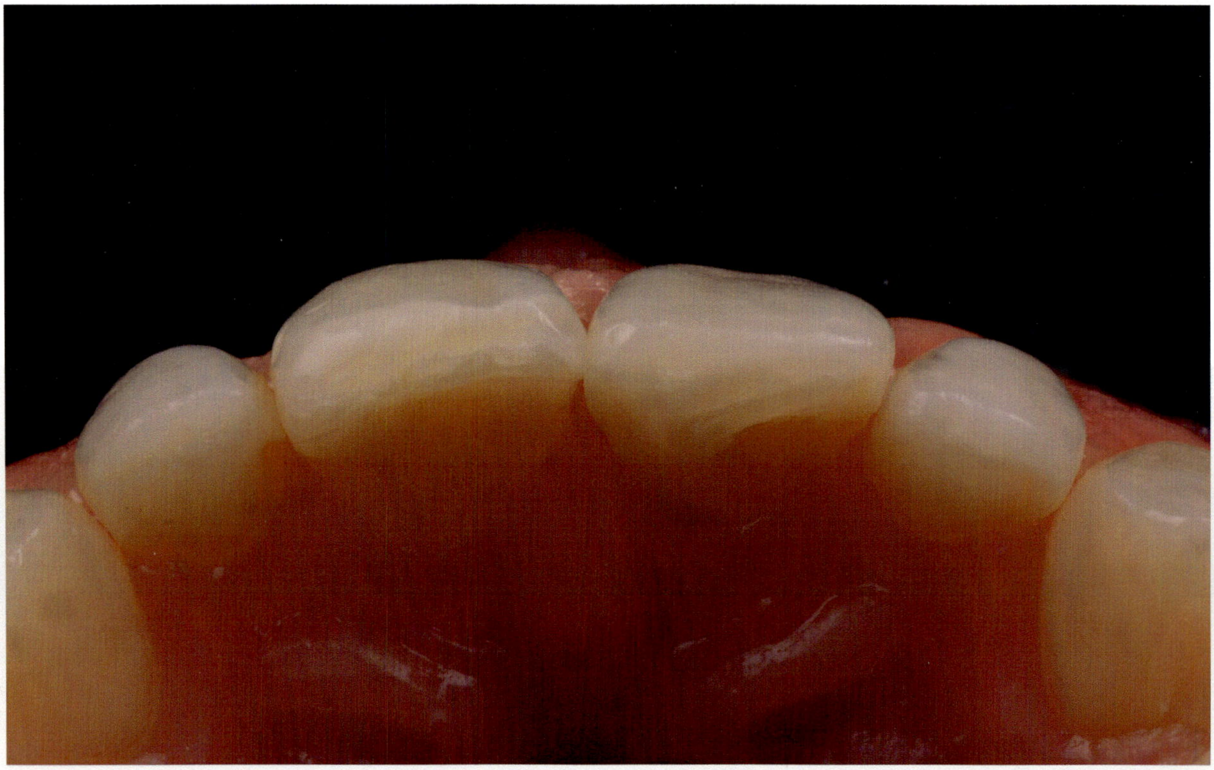

Figure 27 Occlusal view of the restorations.

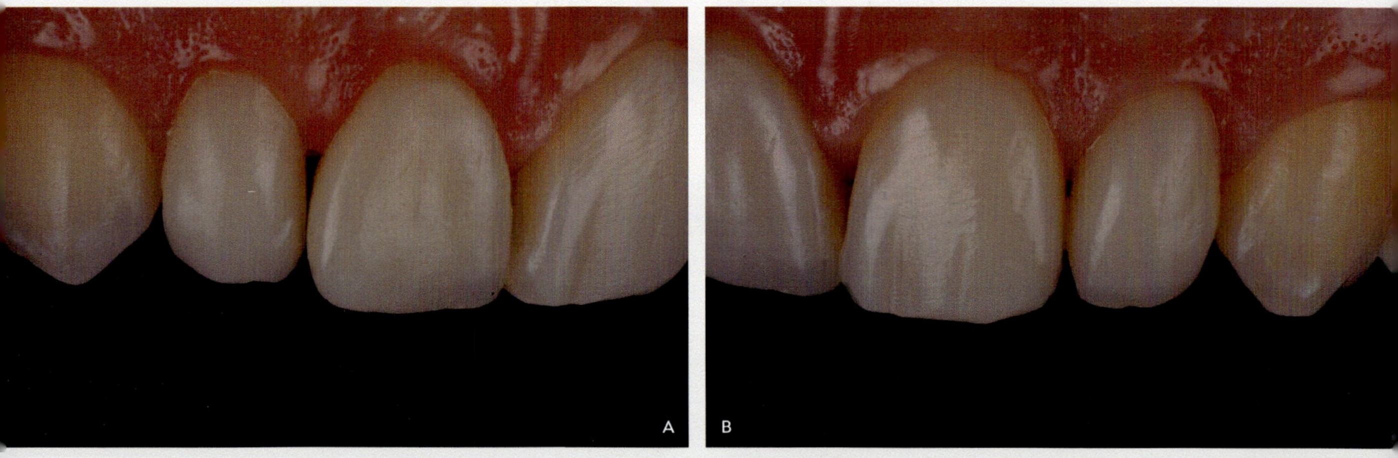

Figures 28a, b Details of the restored quadrants.

CONCLUSIONS

Within its limitations, this technique offers a viable solution for chairside restorations in all cases in which a quick, esthetic, modifiable and repairable solution is required. This technique is especially suitable for young and elderly patients with financial limitations.

Digital planning is easily accessible for the modern dentist and is extremely helpful in solving restorative problems in the anterior area by showing the clinician and the patient an achievable result thus allowing for discussion about the esthetics.

Composite is the material of choice for this kind of technique, thanks to its versatility, stability, and esthetics, even with only two shades[10].

In this case, it's not necessary to use flowable materials, which are too fragile and less esthetically performing over time, just as it's not necessary to warm the paste composite, which risks altering its intrinsic qualities.

In short, this is a user-friendly technique, available to all dentists in any part of the world, in pure StyleItaliano.

BIBLIOGRAPHY

1. Devoto W, Manauta J, Paolone G. IN-OUT: a new concept in composite stratification. *Labline Magazine.* 2013. 3(2):110-127.
2. Magne PC, Douglas WHJ. Additive contour of porcelain veneers: a key element in enamel preservation, adhesion, and esthetics for aging dentition. *The Journal of Adhesive Dentistry.* 1999 Spring;1(1):81-92.
3. Manauta J, Salat A, Monterubbianesi R, Tosco V, Devoto W, Orsini G, Putignano A. Advances in diastema closure and tooth shape change using direct restorations: the Front Wing Technique. *JAED.* 2022 Nov 25;17(4):378-393.
4. Manauta J, Devoto W, Putignano A. I restauri del terzo cervicale: le problematiche dell'interfaccia digitale. *Dental Cadmos.* 2014.
5. Devoto W, Saracinelli M, Manauta J. Composite in everyday dentistry: How to choose the right material and simplify application techniques in the anterior teeth. *JAED.* 2010 Spring;5(1):102-24.
6. Devoto W. Direct and indirect composite restorations in the anterior area: a comparison between the procedures. *QDT yearbook.* 2003;26:127-138.
7. Hardan L, Devoto W, Burgi R, Monteiro P, Zarow M, et al. Immediate dental sealing for adhesive cementation of indirect restorations: a systematic review and meta-analysis. *GELS.* 2022 Mar 11;8(3):175.
8. Hardan L, Burgi R, Cuevas-Suarez CE, Devoto W, Zarow M, Monteiro P, Jakubowicz N, El Zoghbi A, Skaba D, Mancino D, Kharouf N, Haikel Y, Lukomska-Szymanzka M. Effect of different application modalities on the bonding performance of adhesive systems to dentin; a systematic review and meta-analysis. *Cells* [in printing]. 2022.
9. Devoto W, Vanini L. Rifinitura e lucidatura dei restauri in composito. *Il Dentista Moderno, Dossier.* 1999.
10. Paolone G, Orsini G , Manauta J, Devoto W, Putignano A. Composite shade guides and color matching. *IJED.* 2014 Summer;9(2):164-82.

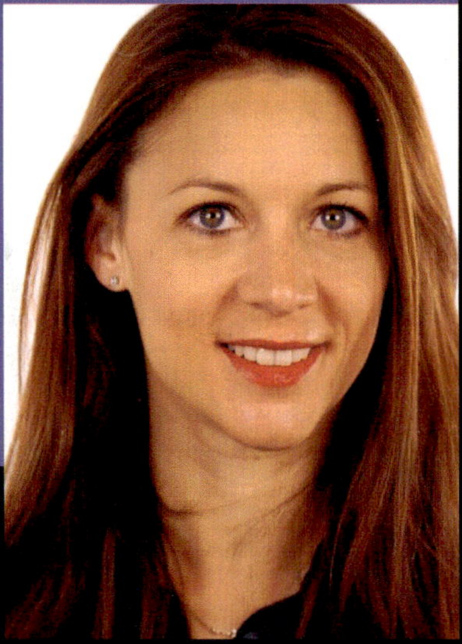

PERRINE BALLAND

France

Dr Balland was born in Nancy (France) 23/05/1981. Former high level athlete in equestrian vaulting, she devoted all her energy to dentistry at the age of 20 when she retired from sports. She graduated from the University of Nancy (France) in 2007.
She continued her studies at the University of New York NYU from 2008 to 2011, where she validated a full time Post-graduate in Periodontology, and won a year fellowship in Cosmetic Dentistry.
Upon her return to France in September 2011, she continued to improve in the field of periodontology in Munich (Germany) with Prs Markus Hurzeler and Otto Zuhr in 2012-2015, and in Florence (Italy) in 2017-2018 with Professors Tonetti and Cortellini through masterclasses.
In recent years, her interest has focused on the use of digital analysis (DSD part 1 in Madrid 2018, DSD part 2 in Sao Paulo 2019 with Dr Christian Coachman, FEEL dentaire formation in Montpellier, France) and adhesive dentistry (StyleItaliano Daily Menu courses 2018 in Santa Margherita Ligure, DCO Formations Lyon 2020), to improve the aesthetics outcome of her periodontal treatments.
Dr Balland has a private practice in Metz (France) and work also in a group practice in Bettembourg (Luxembourg). She is dedicated to periodontics and periodontal plastic surgery exclusively.
She's teaching periodontology for Add Vision dental company in Metz and Strasbourg in France.
She is affiliate to EAED (European Academy of Esthetics Dentistry) since 2019, SFPIO (French Society of Periodontology and Implantology) since 2012 and SNPI (National Syndicate of Periodontology and Implantology) since 2012.
She is a member of editorial board of the dental review NRPI (New Review in Periodontology and Implantology), and she shares her passion with the specialists as a recognized speaker at national (French dental association, orthodontics journey in 2014 and 2016,

At first sight in my exclusive practice as a periodontist, **nothing predestined me to meet StyleItaliano's team, as I wasn't doing any restorative dentistry at the time**. But after a couple of years looking at my cases, I had to face some problems: first, I wasn't entirely satisfied by my management of gingival recession's cases associated with Non-Carious Cervical Lesions (NCCL). In fact, communicating the right position of the maximal line of root coverage (MLRC)[1] to my referent restorative dentists was not easy. The second problem was, for me, to find a solution to help my periodontal patients (after stabilisation) to deal with the "long teeth" aspect and often the black triangles, following periodontal destruction. I had to find a way to keep them motivated to clean, but also to get back self-confidence with some conservative techniques. I wanted to be able to provide them a better aesthetic outcome.
In 2017, I heard about StyleItaliano's courses in a big dental meeting, and I decided to register to their daily menu course edition 34th in Santa Margherita Ligure, on February 2018. Those four days were for me a revelation, giving me some great solutions to be applied for dealing with the perio-restorative interface. Cases you will see below are now my everyday practice dentistry.

A LOOK BACK TO THE PERIO/RESTORATIVE INTERFACE

Modern dentistry techniques have improved human dentition with increased longevity of teeth through improved personal oral hygiene, fluoridation, and advanced restorative procedure[2,3]. However, performing thorough daily oral hygiene for extended periods in association with erosive aggressions, and tooth flexure will invariably wear the tooth substance away from a cement-enamel area (the neck of the tooth) and induce cervical non-carious cervical lesions (NCCLs)[3]. Gingival consequences (*e.g.*, gingival recession) of aggressive personal oral hygiene procedures also have been described[4]. Open gingival embrasures or black triangles are also noticeably unesthetic and negatively affect the smile. They facilitate retention of food debris which can negatively affect the health of the periodontium[5]. **Black triangles are present in more than one third of all adults but are more frequent in adult patients who suffer bone loss**[6]. The treatment plan should be discussed with patients before starting dental treatment. Its management varies depending on the etiological factor, but is favourably managed by a team usually including restorative and periodontal surgical treatment[7].

The main indications for the treatment of gingival recessions are aesthetic concern, root hypersensitivity, prevention or management of root caries and cervical abrasion, enhancement of restorative outcomes and facilitation of plaque control efforts.
The development of non-carious cervical lesions (NCCL) may occur on exposed root surfaces due to various mechanisms such as corrosion, stress forces, and friction[8]. Main concerns related to the association between gingival recessions and root abrasion are aesthetic concerns, dentin hypersensitivity, root caries/demineralization and bacterial plaque accumulation, which are the main indications for the treatment[9]. Because of the multiple factors involved, such as disappearance of the cemento-enamel junction (CEJ) and the depth and the width of the cervical lesions, treatment of gingival recession associated with an NCCL could not be easy and predictable. Therefore, to solve all these problems, a combined surgical/restorative therapy was proposed for treatment of these combined defects[10,11].

Frequently, when treating the aesthetic concerns of the patient, practitioners focus on the teeth (the white) and ignore the gingiva (the pink). Yet, both these aspects need to be addressed to provide the best aesthetic outcome and to correct what is either naturally present or the result of wear and tear over the years. It is not unusual to restore the anterior maxillary teeth with direct resin veneers, porcelain veneers, or full-coverage crowns, and end up with a patient who may not be completely satisfied with the result. This is often on a subconscious level, and the patient and practitioner cannot pinpoint what doesn't "look right".

The best analogy to explain this: **even the most beautiful picture needs a frame to do it justice**. When restoring the maxillary anterior teeth, we need to regard the gingival tissue as the frame for the teeth to be restored. Adjusting the gingival margins to make the central incisors appear even, to get the zeniths of the anterior teeth in harmony, should all be considered before proceeding with the restoration of the teeth.

Restoration of non-carious cervical lesions with resin composites[12] is one of the treatment options since a long term, but the retention of the restorations located at the crown-root junction used to be a cause of clinical concern. In fact, in the past[13] we did not rely as much as now on adhesion to the tooth structures via adhesive systems, also esthetic was not as close to nature as it is today. Shrinkage during polymerization used to be an important shortcoming of composite restorations, leading to bonding failure and dental and periodontal consequences[14,15].

Restorative materials must be biocompatible to minimize their adverse effects on periodontal tissues induced by direct contact. Resin composites or resin-modified glass ionomer cements have been commonly used to restore NCCLs. Resin-ionomer materials have many properties such as biocompatibility with soft and hard tissues and displaying high marginal adaptation and minimal surface roughness, as well as allowing them to be used successfully in the subgingival region. Composite resin materials have many advantages including aesthetics and surface characteristics in terms of finishing and polishing[16,17]. It has been reported that well-adapted and finished composite resins seem have no adverse effects on the periodontal margin.

Clinical Case 1

Upper and Lower arch treatment
Periodontal and restorative treatment

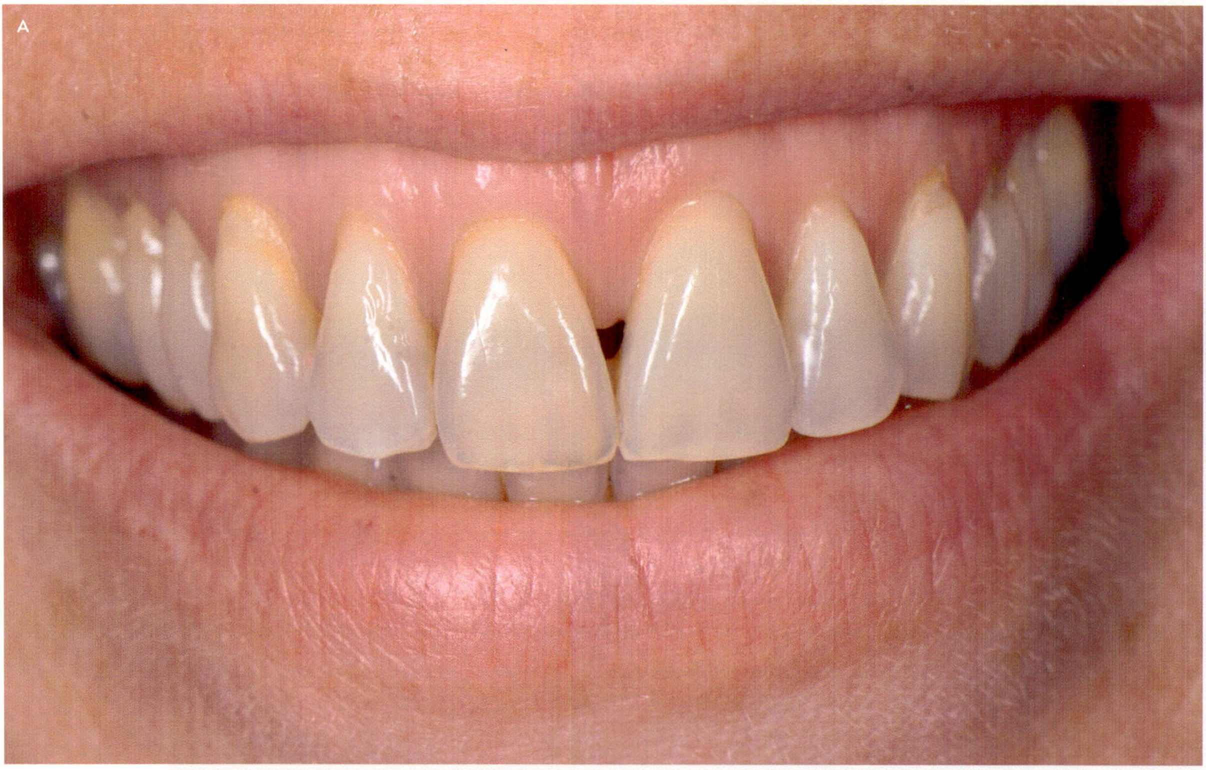

Figures 1a, b, c 51-years-old female patient complaining about root hypersensitivity and the huge black triangle between 11 and 21, associated with a gummy smile. She got through orthodontic treatment five years before and she had some restorative class V composites by her dentist to reduce hypersensitivity.

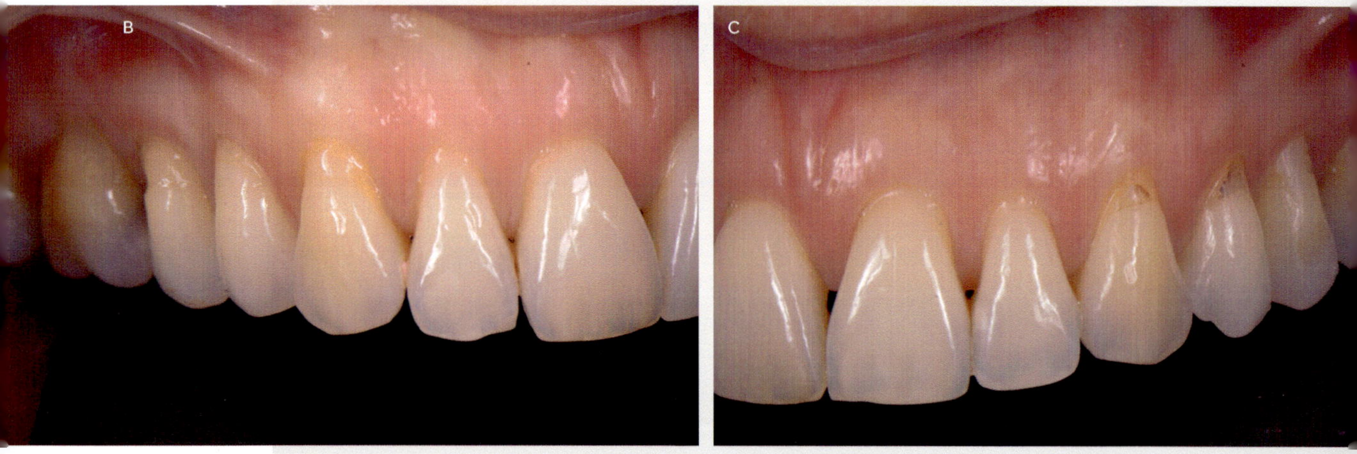

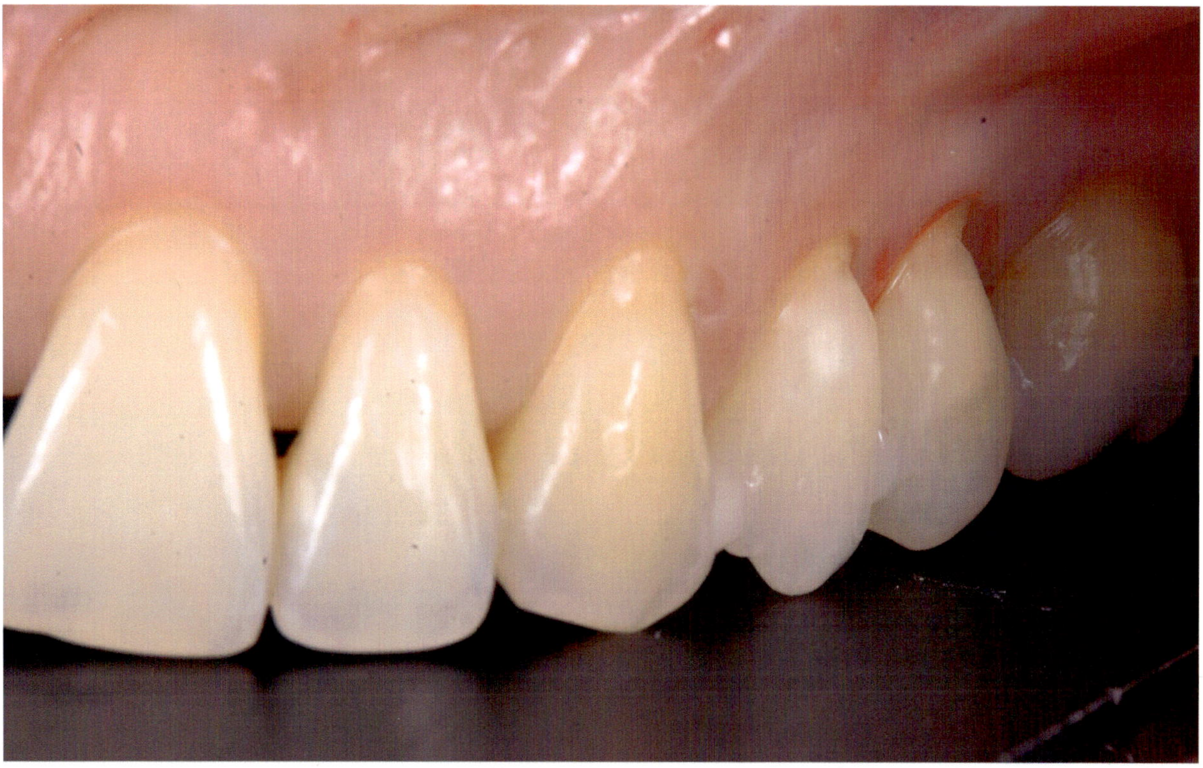

Figure 2 Day of surgery; first step was to remove the previous restoratives fillings which were colonizing the root surface, and to redo the estimated cement-enamel junction to the maximal line of root coverage (MLRC) describe by Zucchelli et al[1]. I also had to do some interdental composites in spots to hold my double cross sling sutures (ZUHR)[21].

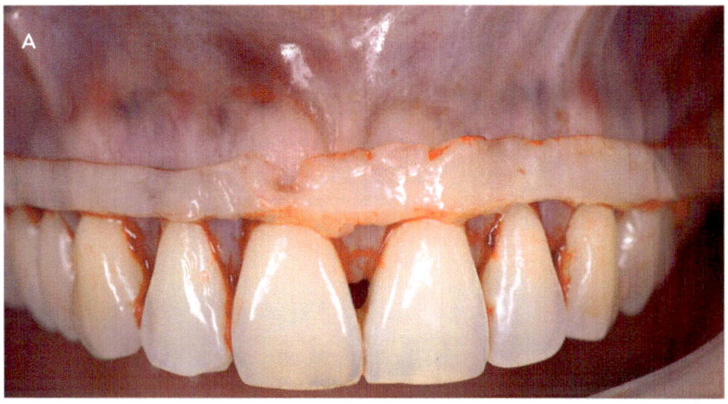

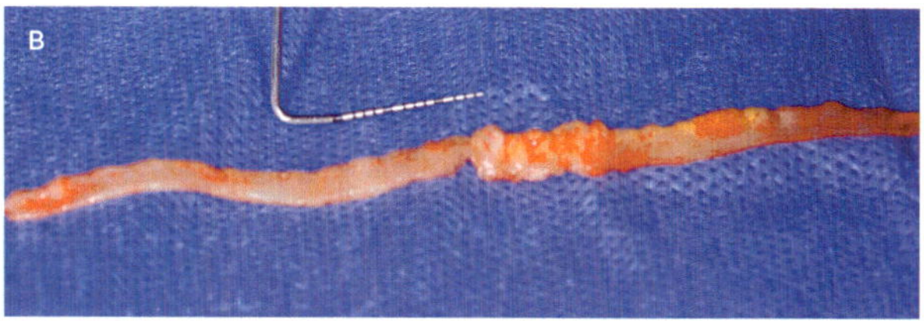

Figure 3a, b Harvest a small band of free gingival graft deepithelialized from mesial of 17 to mesial of 27 for root coverage using a tunnel technique.

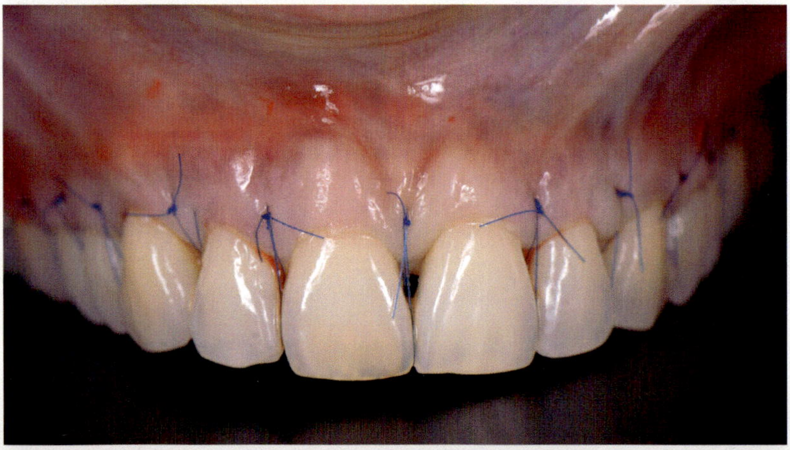

Figure 4a Double cross sling sutures at the end of surgery.

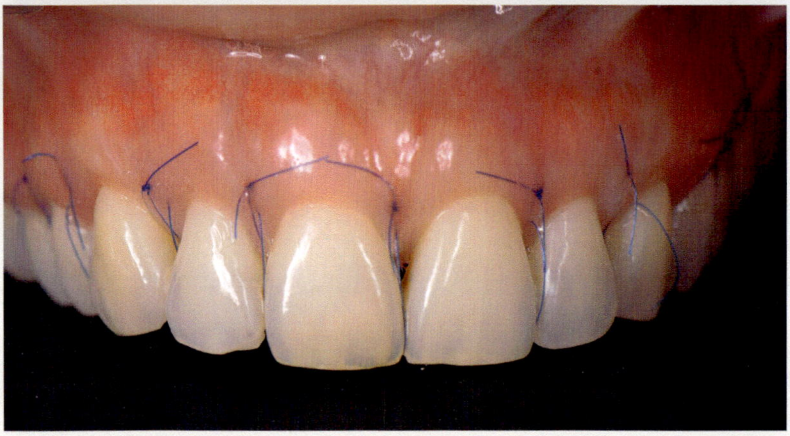

Figure 4b Follow-up at 15 days.

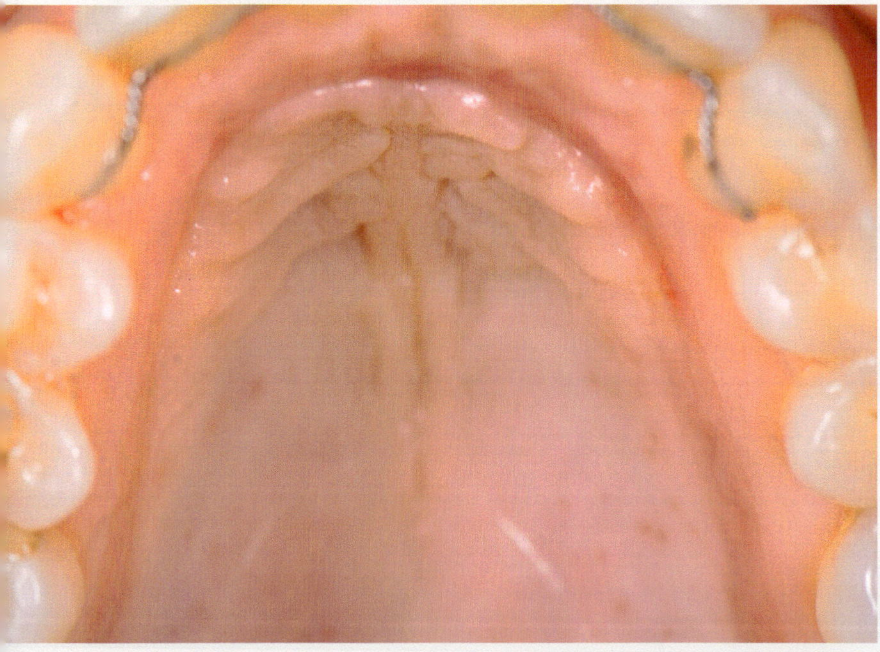

Figure 5 15 days follow-up of the palatal donor site. The patient was wearing a palatal protection plaque for 5 days. An hemostatic sponge was used, no sutures.

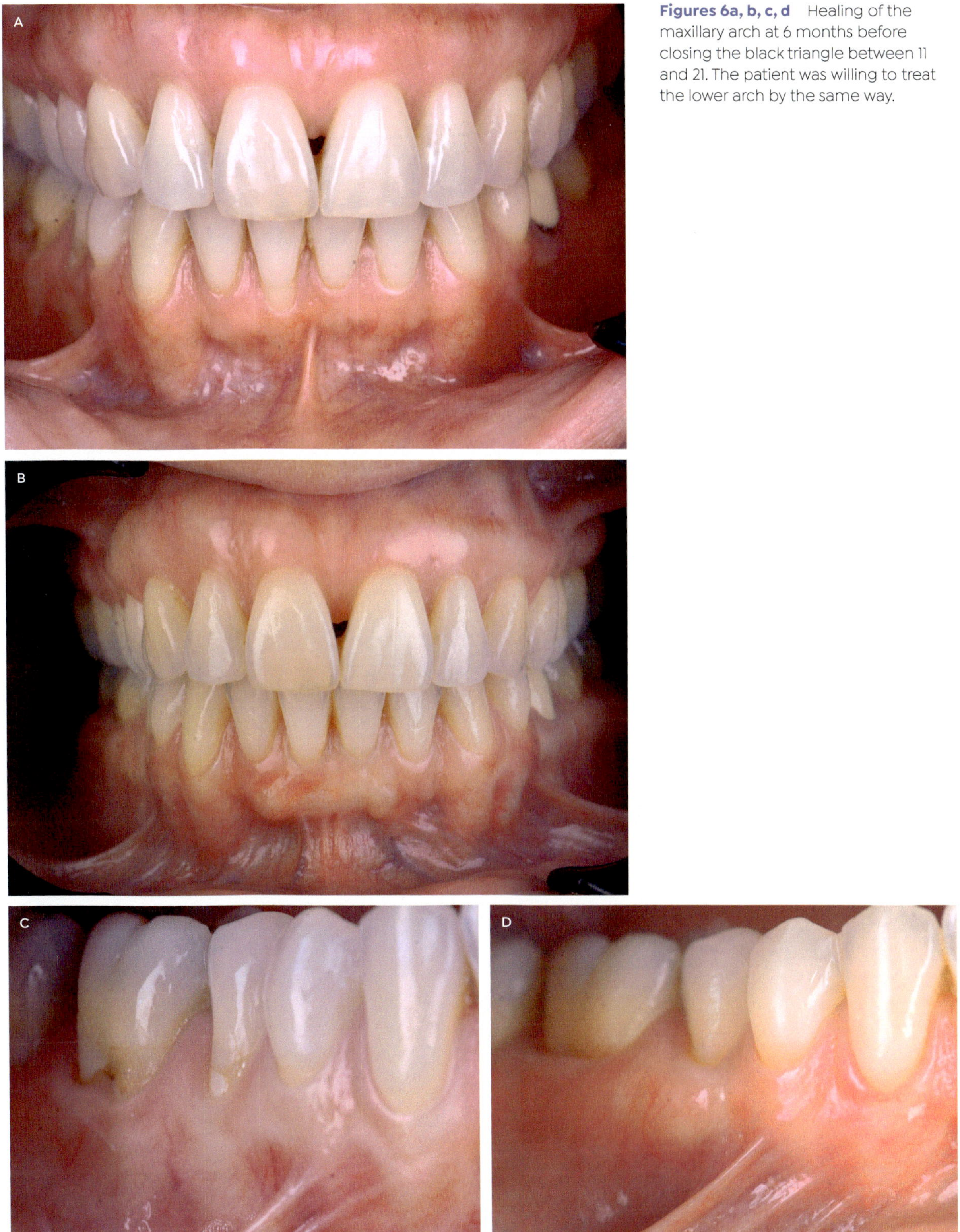

Figures 6a, b, c, d Healing of the maxillary arch at 6 months before closing the black triangle between 11 and 21. The patient was willing to treat the lower arch by the same way.

Figure 7 Frontal face view and smile of the patient at 1 year before closing the black triangle 11/21.

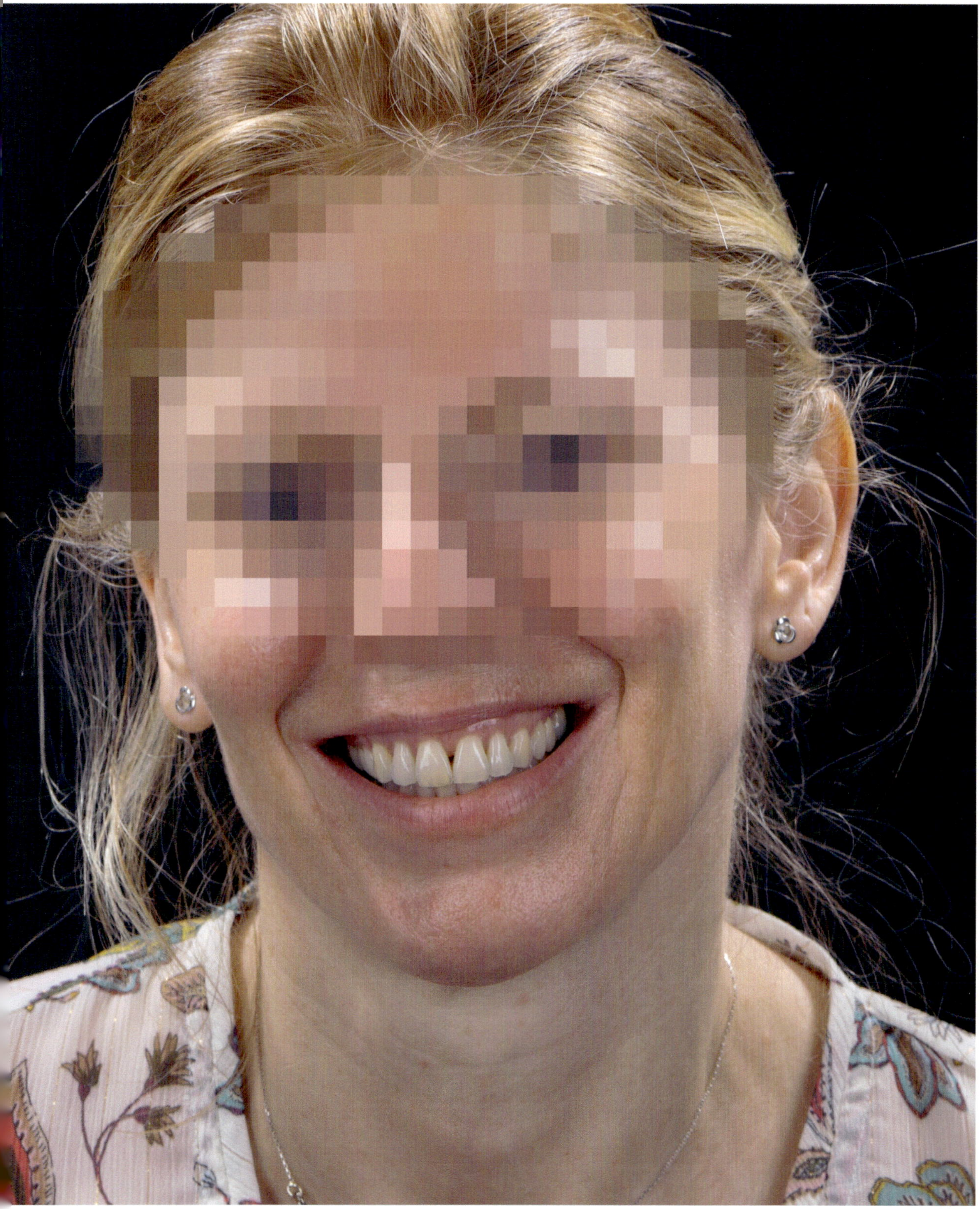

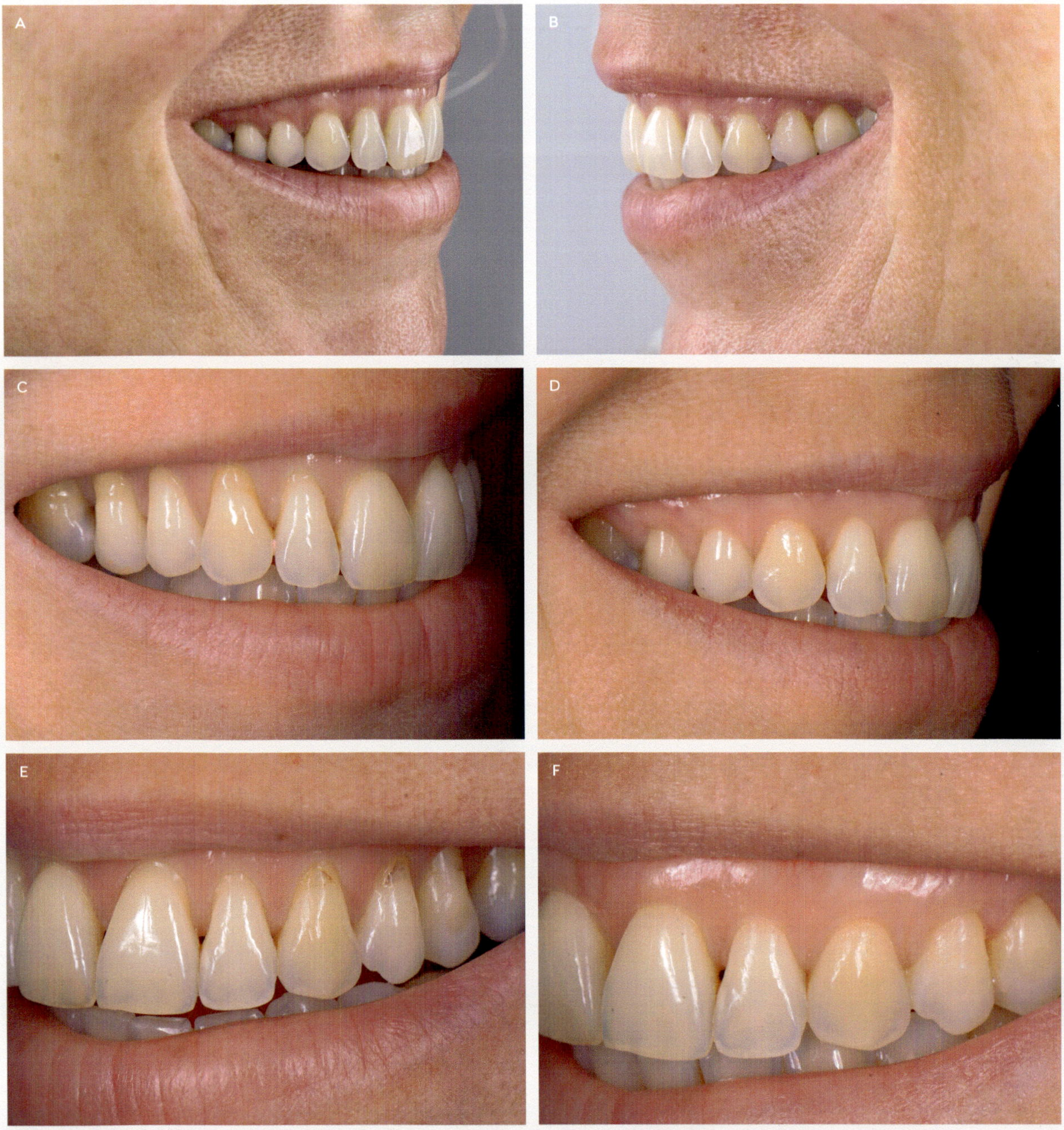

Figure 8a, b, c, d, e, f Lateral face views and smile of the patient at 3 years post periodontal and restorative approach of the maxillary arch treating recessions and non cervical carious lesions (NCCL).

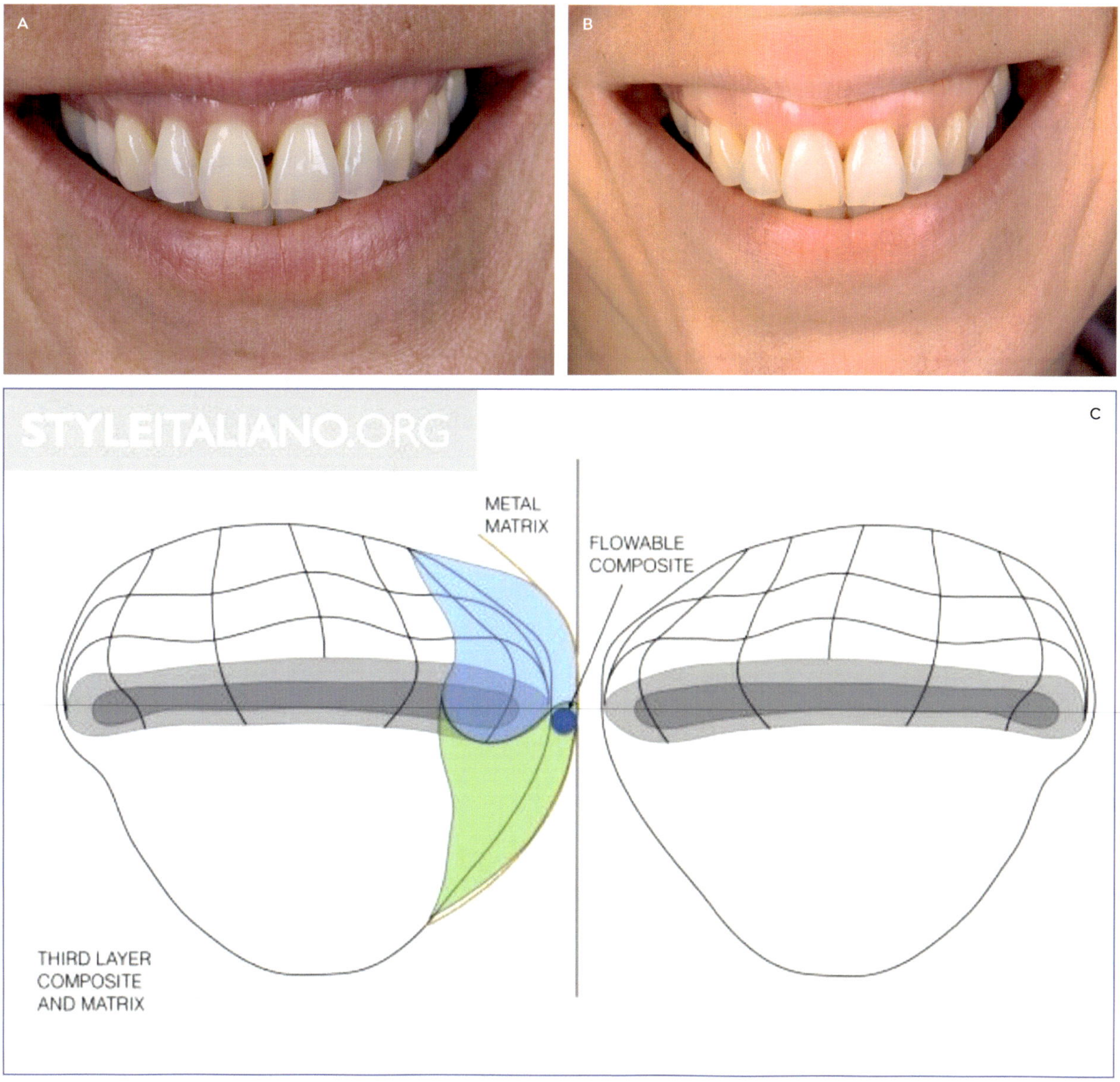

Figure 9a, b, c Closing the black triangle between 11/21.

Clinical Case 2

Upper and Lower arch treatment
Periodontal
and restorative treatment

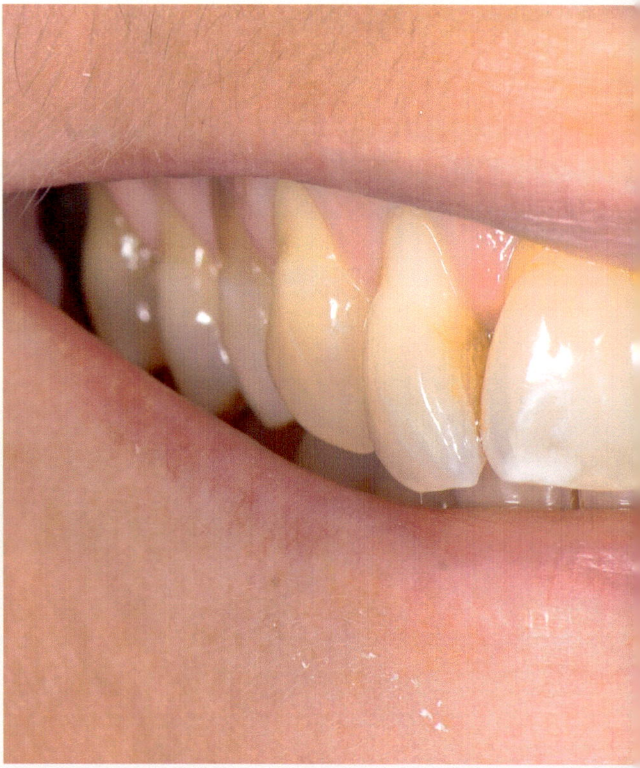

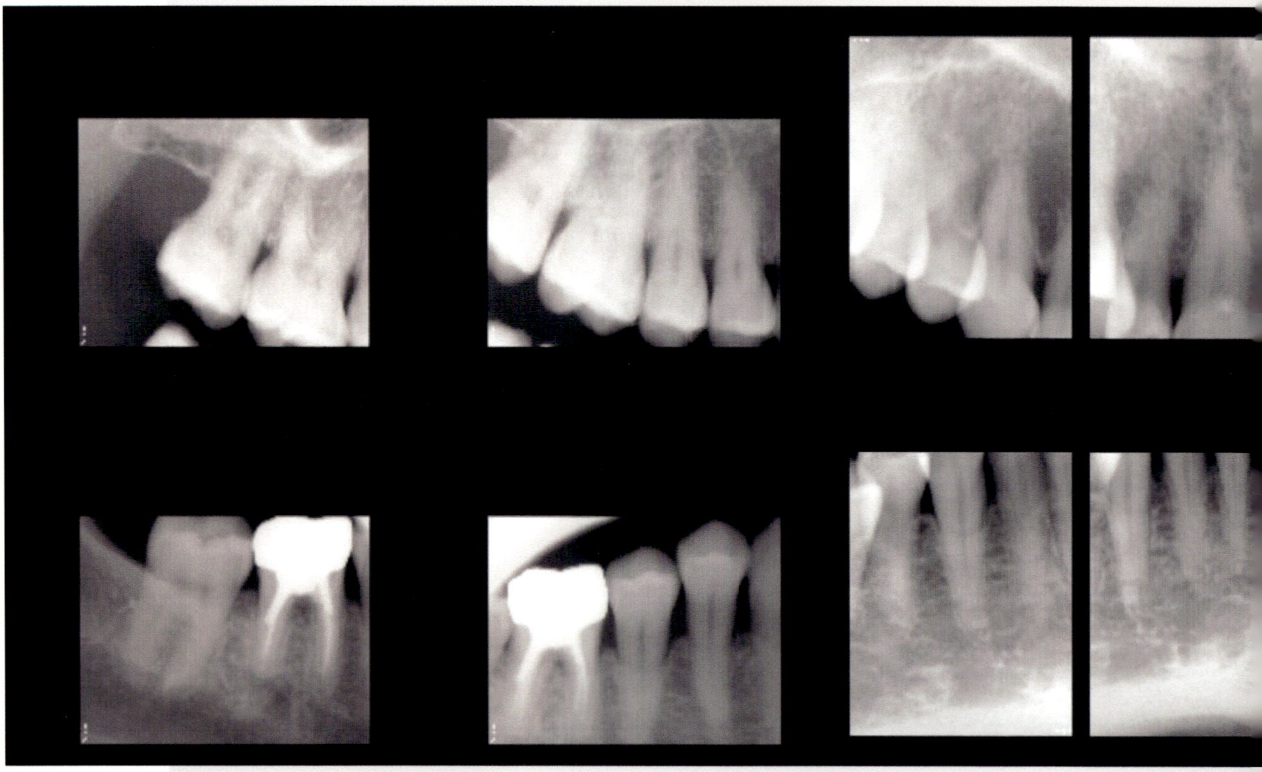

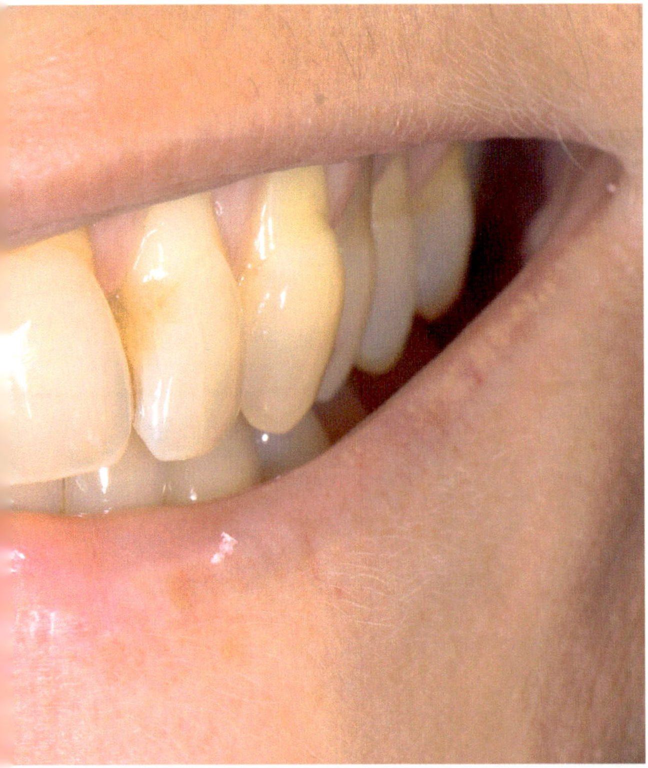

Figure 1 Smile view of a 49-years-old female patient. She had a non-surgical periodontal treatment 5 years before, to treat her localized periodontitis stage 1 grade A. Secondary migrations can be observe on teeth 12 and 22. The patient is now stable and would like to get some solutions to get a better esthetics outcome. Her chief complain was «I can see my roots by smiling and I have a lot of hypersensitivity».

Figure 2 Radiographic status 5 years after periodontal treatment.

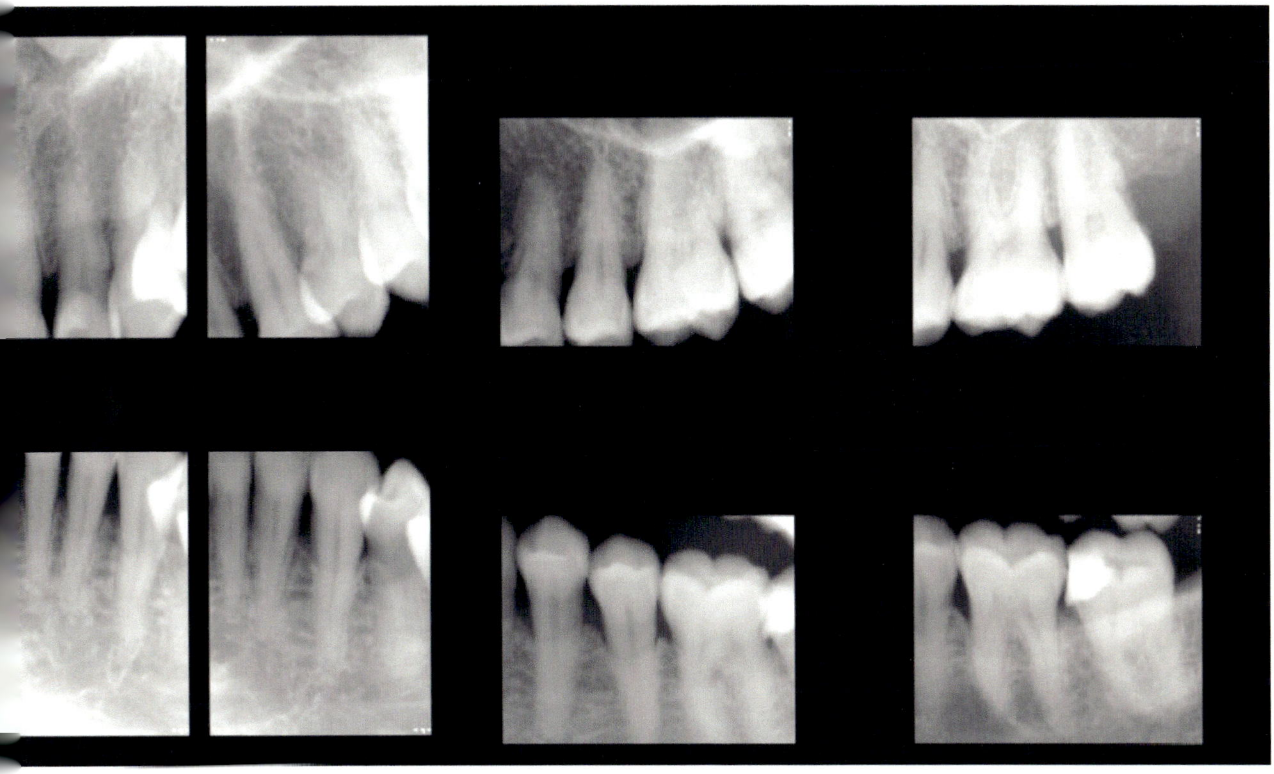

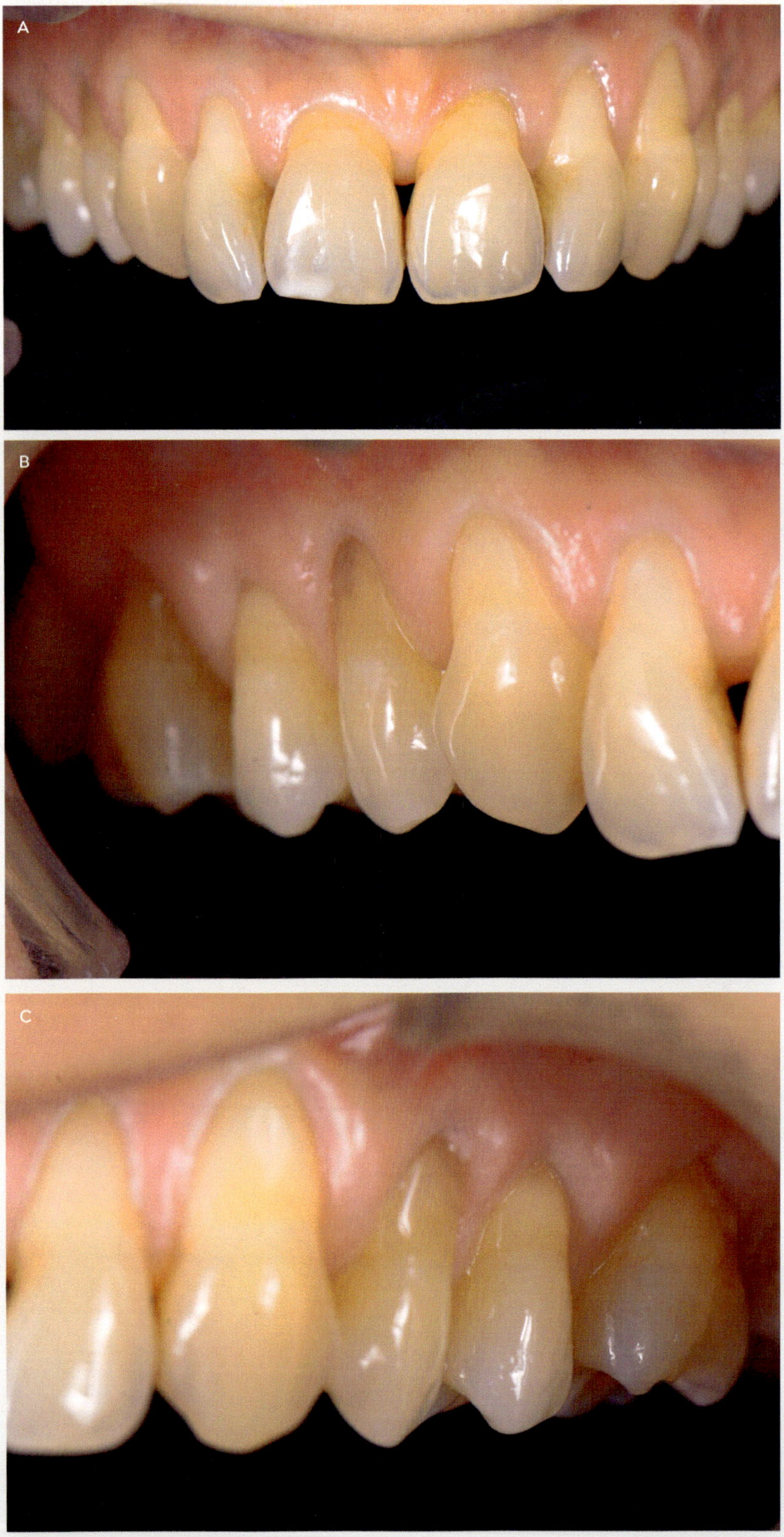

Figures 3a, b, c Intraoral facial and lateral view pictures.

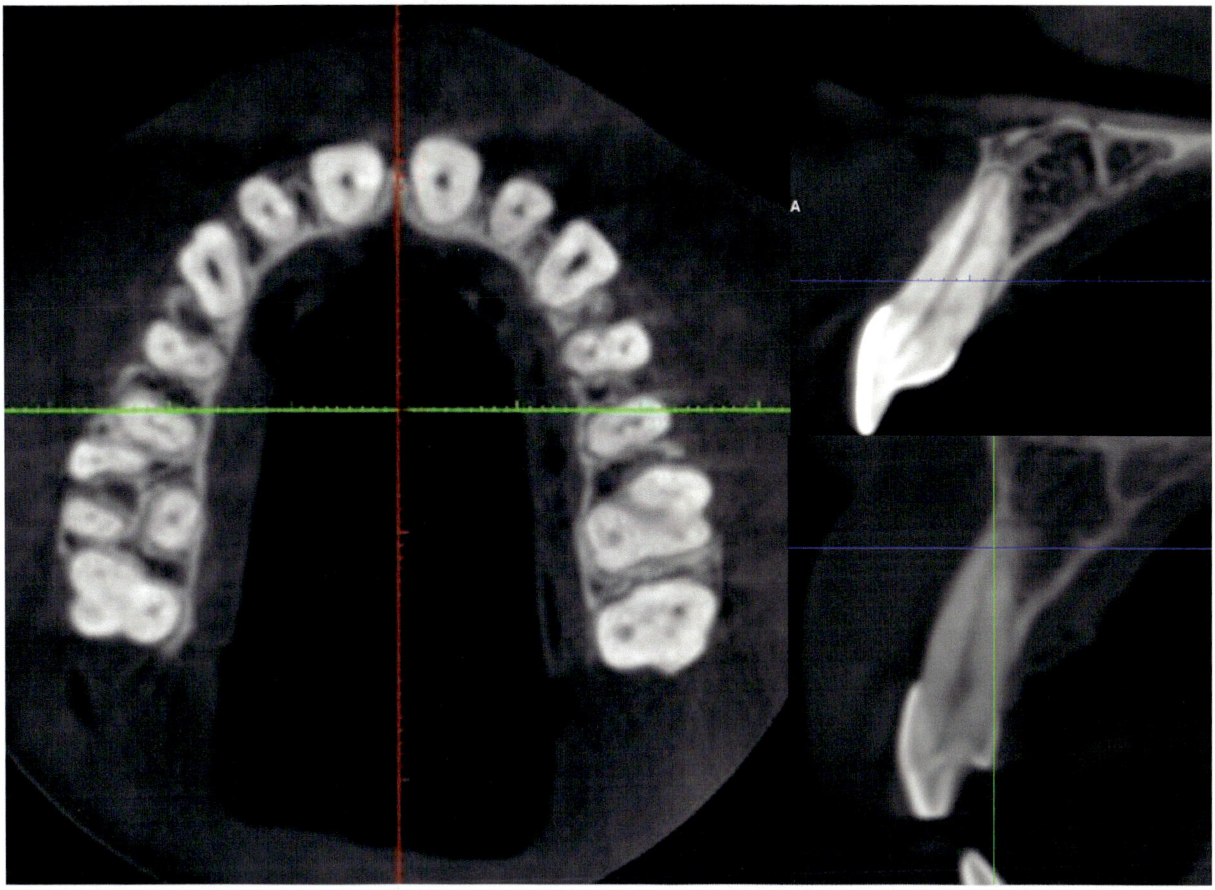

Figures 4a, b, c 3D-cone beam view of the maxillary arch. Almost Half of the roots are out of the bone crest. The orthodontist refused to do a treatment, he said it was too risky, we could damage more of the periodontium. So I had to think about the case differently using restorative and periodontal muco gingival surgery to solve the case.

OPTIONS

Restorative Therapy

Zucchelli G, Testori T, De Sanctis M.
Clinical and anatomical factors limiting treatment outcomes of gingival recession: A new method to predetermine the line of root coverage.
J Periodontol. 2006;77:714-721.

Orthodontic Therapy

Laursen MG, Rylev M, Melsen B.
The role of orthodontics in the repair of gingival recessions.
Am J Orthod Dentofacial Orthop. 2020;157(1):29-34.

100% of root coverage is not possible

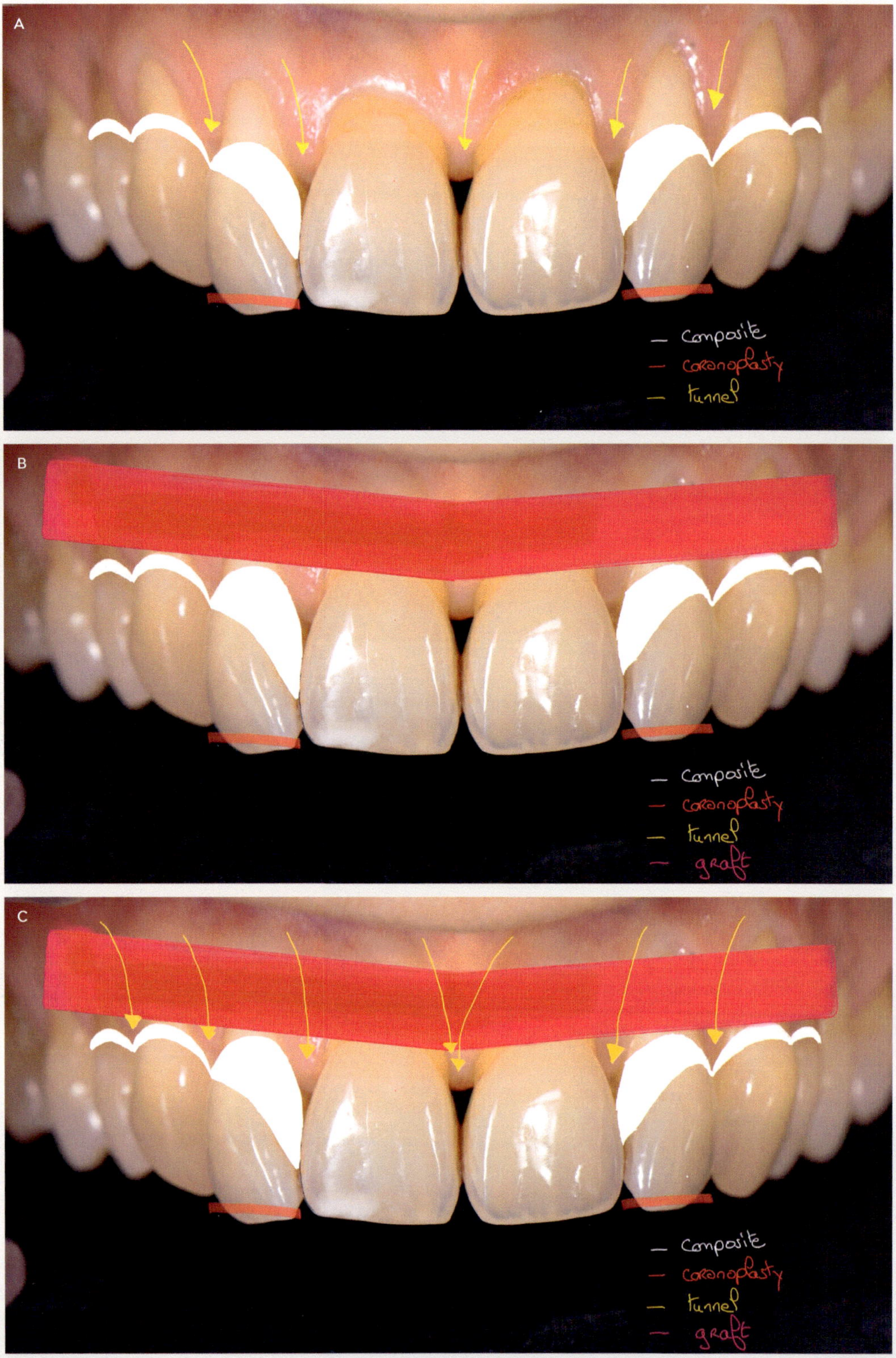

Figures 5a, b, c Restorative part: doing a coronoplasty on the incisal edge of 12 and 22. Reshaping 12 and 22 with Composites. Recreating the maximal line of root coverage on the collar of teeth 13, 14, 23, 24 to guide soft tissue healing of my graft.

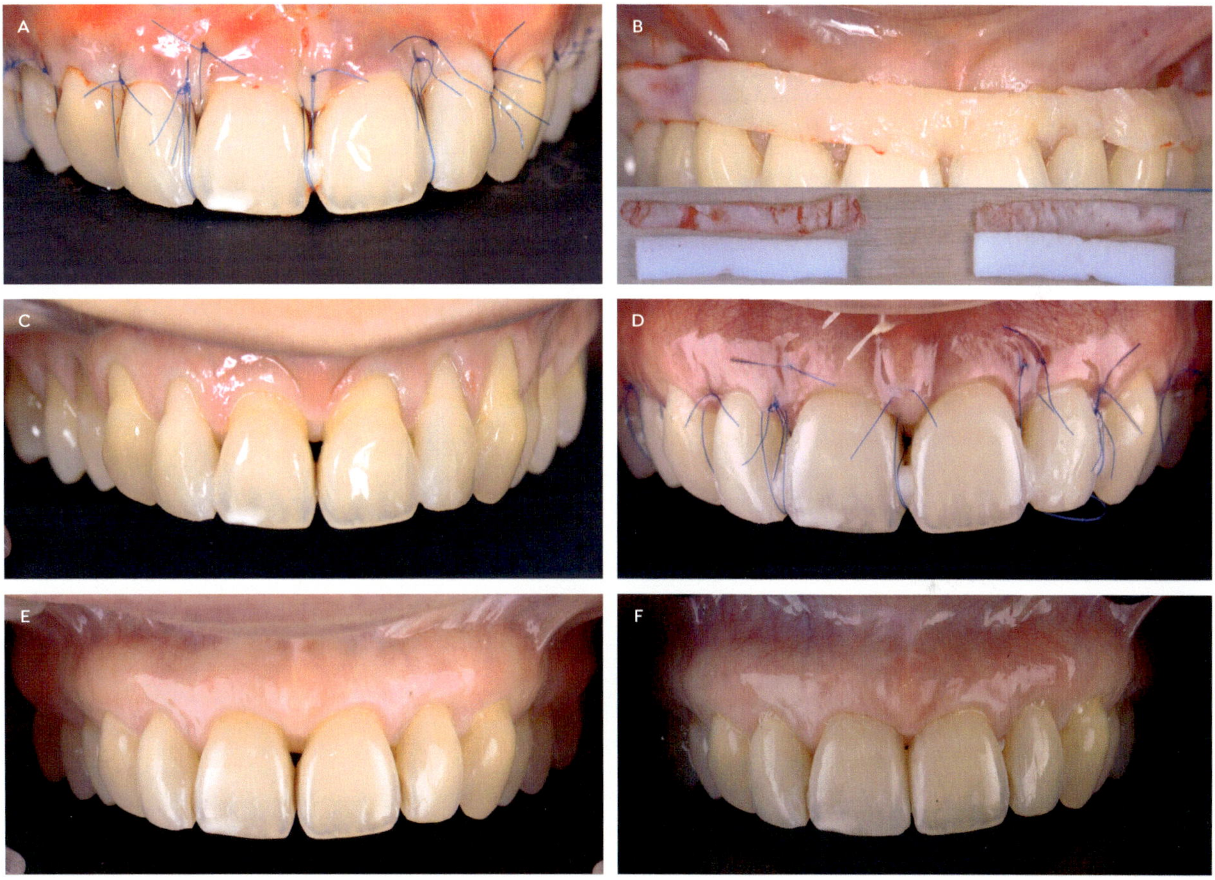

Figures 6a, b, c, d, e, f Surgical part: connective tissue graft harvested from both side of the palate, using a tunnel technique and a double cross sling suture technique to get maximum root coverage. Healing at 15 days was good. Then I waited 6 months to use the front wing technique to close the black triangles between 11 and 21.

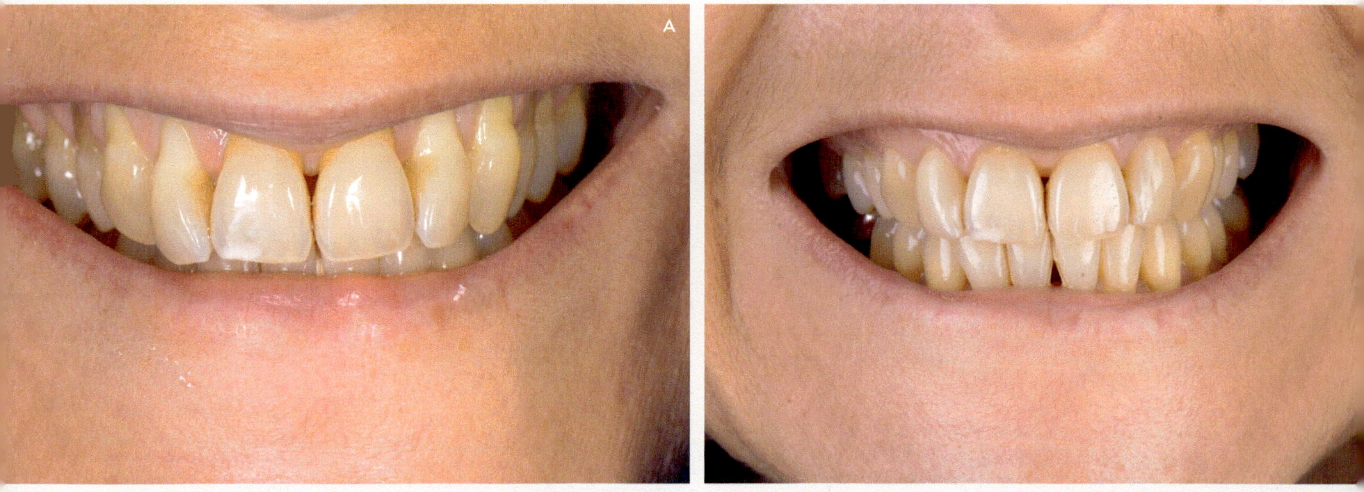

Figures 7a, b, c
a. Initial smile view
b. Healing at 6 months
c. Gealing at 18 month post surgical and restorative phase

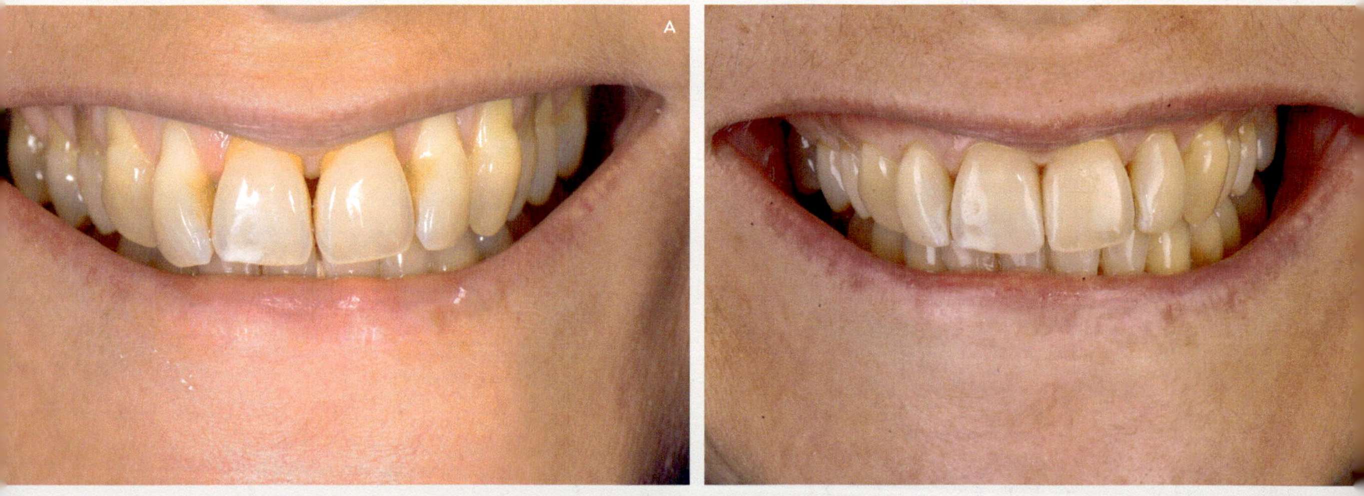

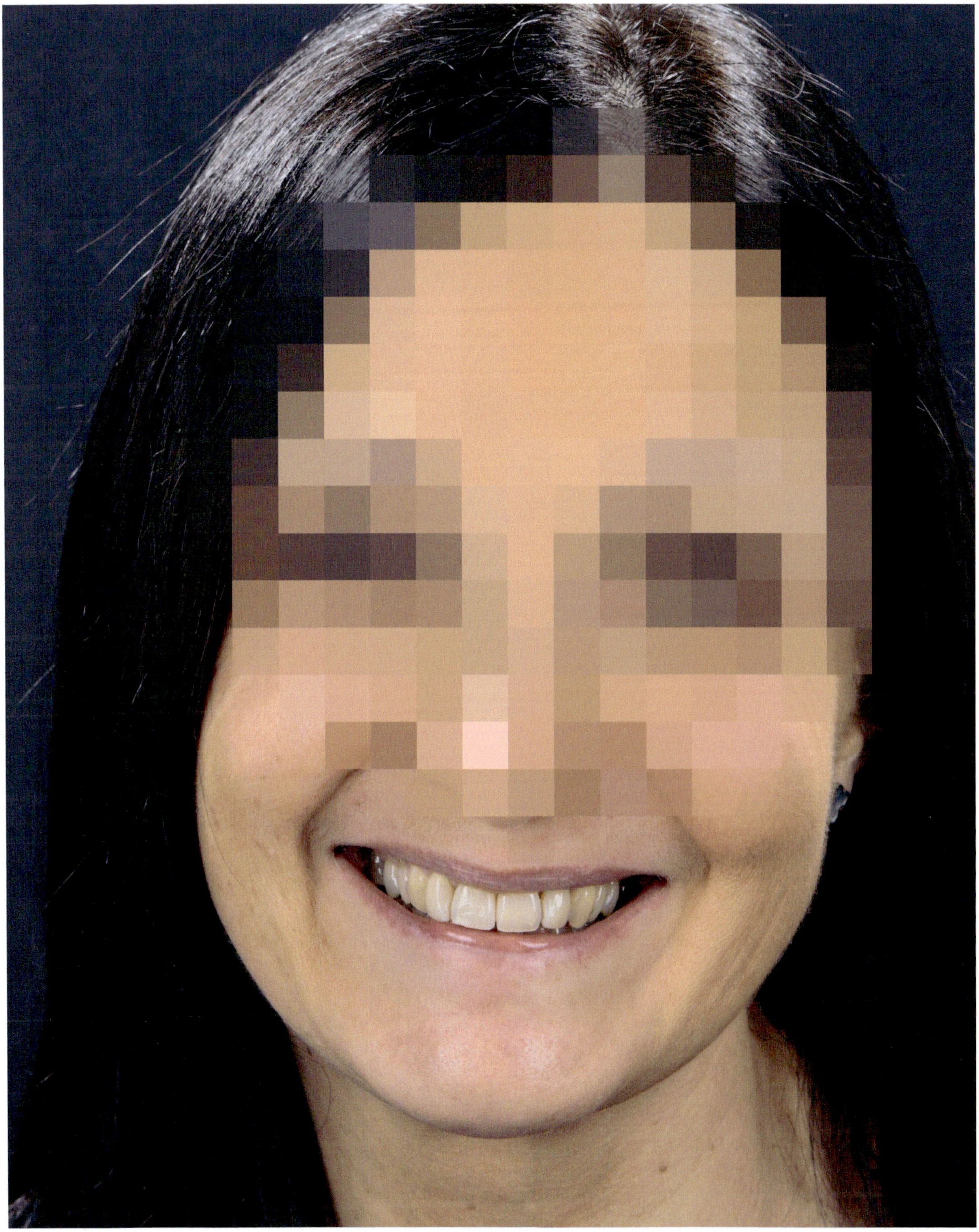

Figure 8 Face view of an happy patient who benefited from a combine approach of surgical and restorative therapy.

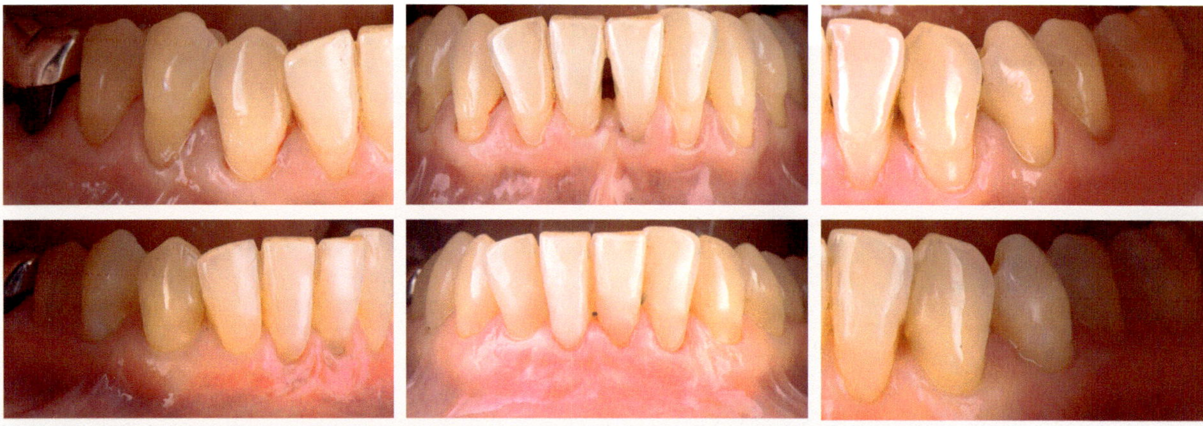

Figures 9a, b, c, d, e, f Two years after the maxillary arch treatment, this patient came back to ask for the same treatment approach on the lower arch. Follow-up at 18 months.

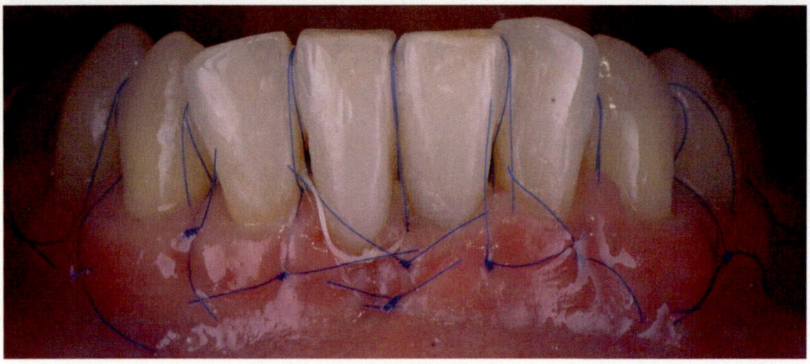

Figure 10 Surgery day.

BIBLIOGRAPHY

1. Zucchelli G, Mele M, Stefanini M, Mazzotti C, Mounssif I, Marzadori M, Montebugnoli L Predetermination of root coverage. *J Periodontol.* 2010 Jul;81(7):1019-26.
2. Bartlett DW, Shah P. A critical review of non-carious cervical (wear) lesions and the role of abfraction, erosion, and abrasion. *J Dent Res.* 2006;85:306-312.
3. Grippo JO. Noncarious cervical lesions: the decision to ignore or restore. *J. Esthet. Dent.* 4(Suppl), 55-64 (1992).
4. Heasman PA, Holliday R, Bryant A & Preshaw PM. Evidence for the occurrence of gingival recession and non-carious cervical lesions as a consequence of traumatic toothbrushing. *J. Clin. Periodontol.* 42(Suppl 16), S237-255 (2015).
5. Van der Geld P, Oosterveld P, Van Heck G, Kuijpers-Jagtman AM. Smile attractiveness. Self-perception and influence on personality. *Angle Orthod.* 2007;77:759-65.
6. Tarnow DP, Magner AW, Fletcher P. The effect of the distance from the contact point to the crest of bone on the presence or absence of the interproximal dental papilla. *J Periodontol.* 1992;63(12):995-996.
7. Chambrone L, Tatakis DN. Periodontal soft tissue root coverage procedures: a systematic review from the AAP regeneration workshop. *J Periodontol.* 2015;86:S8-S51.
8. Bartlett DW, Shah P. A critical review of non-carious cervical (wear) lesions and the role of abfraction, erosion, and abrasion. *J Dent Res.* 2006;85:306-312.
9. Zucchelli G, Gori G, Mele M. Non-carious cervical lesions associated with gingival recessions: a decision-making process. *J Periodontol.* 2011;82:1713-1724.
10. Lucchesi JA, Santos VR, Amaral CM, Peruzzo DC, Duarte PM. Coronally positioned flap for treatment of restored root surfaces: a 6-month clinical evaluation. *J Periodontol.* 2007;78:615-623.
11. Santamaria MP, et al. Resin composite plus connective tissue graft to treat single maxillary gingival recession associated with non-carious cervical lesion: randomized clinical trial. *J. Clin. Periodontol.* 43, 461-468 (2016).

CONCLUSIONS

Nowadays with the evolution of all the materials, combining surgical/restorative approaches was observed as safe, predictable and effective as the surgical procedures alone[18,19]. A randomized-controlled clinical trial[20] has reported that this approach could provide soft tissue coverage without damage to periodontal tissues in the treatment of gingival recessions associated with NCCL.

Back to 2018, in StyleItaliano's course, you can easily imagine that I was the only periodontist there. The team on site, Walter Devoto, Angelo Putigano and Jordi P Manauta, really took some time with me during the hands on, and gave me several exercises and tips to work on for my specific interest with the techniques of closing diastemas, black triangles and treating class V lesion with composites. Of course, taking the learning curve back to my practice was not that easy, but I perseverated and I will continue in this direction.

I am very grateful to StyleItaliano which really change my way of treating periodontal patients. I don't think we heard the last of this "PINK/WHITE" interface power.

12. Perez CDR, et al. Restoration of non-carious cervical lesions: when, why, and how. *Int J Dent.* 2012.
13. Paolantonio M, D'ercole S, Perinetti G. Clinical and microbiological effects of different restorative materials on the periodontal tissues adjacent to subgingival class V restorations. *J Clin Periodontol.* 2004;31:200-207.
14. Duquia, Rde. C, Osinaga, PW, Demarco FF, de V Habekost L & Conceição EN. Cervical microleakage in MOD restorations: in vitro comparison of indirect and direct composite. *Oper. Dent.* 2006;31:682-687.
15. Gonçalves F, Kawano Y & Braga RR. Contraction stress related to composite inorganic content. *Dent. Mater. Off. Publ. Acad. Dent. Mater.2010*;26:704-709.
16. Manauta J, Salat A, Putignano A, Devoto W, Paolone G, Hardan LS. Stratification in anterior teeth using one dentine shade and a predefined thickness of enamel: a new concept in composite layering—Part II. *Odontostomatol Trop.* 2014 Sep;37(147):5-13.
17. Manauta J, Salat A, Putignano A, Devoto W, Villares CF, Hardan LS. Natural, polarized light and the choice of composite: a key to success in shade matching of direct anterior restorations—Part II. *Odontostomatol Trop.* 2016 Dec;39(156):5-15.
18. Zucchelli G, Gori G, Mele M. Non-carious cervical lesions associated with gingival recessions: a decision- making process. *J Periodontol.* 2011;82:1713-1724.
19. Zucchelli G, Testori T, DeSanctis M. Clinical and anatomical factors limiting treatment outcomes of gingival recession: A new method to predetermine the line of root coverage. *J Periodontol* 2006;77:714-721.
20. Santamaria MP, Queiroz LA, Mathias IF. Resin composite plus connective tissue graft to treat single maxillary gingival recession associated with non-carious cervical lesion: randomized clinical trial. *J Clin Periodontol.* 2016;43:461-46.
21. Zuhr O, Rebele SF, Thalmair T, Fickl S, Hürzeler MB. A modified suture technique for plastic periodontal and implant surgery—the double crossed suture. *Eur J Esthet Dent.* 2009 Winter;4(4):338-47.

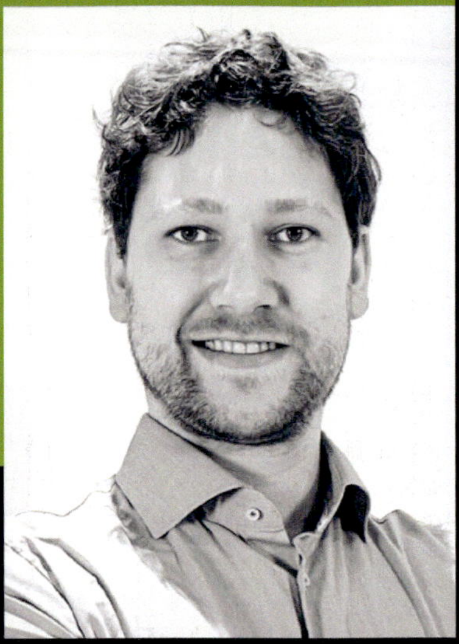

VALENTIN VERVACK

Belgium

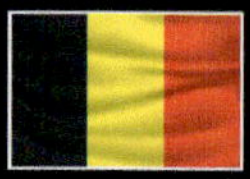

Valentin Vervack graduated in Science of Dentistry from Ghent University (Belgium) in 2013. After his Bachelor and Master' degrees, he started working in his fathers' private practice but also stayed active at Ghent University for research and mentoring.
In 2017 he and his wife took over the private clinic and he started focusing more on esthetic, adhesive and microscope enhanced dentistry.
In 2018, Vervack was one of the winners of the StyleItaliano Bulk One contest and, since then, he kept close contacts with the group.
In 2020, he started as a silver member at StyleItaliano. During these years, Vervack kept busy at Ghent University with clinical and in vitro studies, entering a PhD program in 2017, with "the full digital workflow for single tooth restorations" as a subject.
In 2021, together with 3 colleagues, he founded the "Dental Bootcamp" continuous education platform, which focusses on hands-on centered innovating dental courses.
Vervack has published several papers on specialized journals and he has been lecturing in national and international congresses and events on restorative and digital dentistry.

COLORIMETRY ENHANCED SHADE MATCHING, USING A PREDICTABLE LAYERING AND FINISHING TECHNIQUE FOR THE SINGLE CENTRAL INCISOR

Recreating the perfect symmetry in shape, surface gloss, texture, and – last but far from least important – shade matching is challenging. Shade and shape are the two main pillars which determine the success of anterior restorations. Even if only one of them is imperfect, the other will not be able to compensate for it, even in seemingly simple cases. Well described protocols for shaping, finishing, and polishing make it feasible to sculp the shape. Although multilayer composite has been around for a very long time, the success has always been depending on the experience of the operator with a specific composite systems[1]. When looking at the first figures, every dentist will immediately have figured out a composite recipe to restore this tooth with their trusted composite system. The problem remains that no standard, reproducible protocol is available to restore the tooth shade within clinically acceptable terms. The most common method is a visual verification, by comparing a shade guide to the dentition. Due to a large diversity in shade guides and composite systems the shade matching is challenging[2]. Digital colorimeters can help to facilitate the reproducibility and to better understand the shade mixtures of a tooth. In this case, a precise colorimetric analysis of the neighboring tooth was performed through the Optishade colorimeter. This results in a detailed shade-mapping in the shade guide-library of choice (e.g., Vita, Vita 3D-master).

DISCUSSION AND CLINICAL CASE

The measurements and colorimetric results for the case presented in 1, 2 can be found in 3. A dual layering recipe was chosen, as it is the most predictable and feasible one. A single mass technique would not match the shade close enough and a multi-layer approach is time- and energy-consuming and less predictable. For the most palatal layer, a chromatic dentin shade was chosen (A2D), while for the "enamel" layer, a more translucent shade with less chroma was selected (WB). This was created and matched by using the My Shade Guide technique[4].

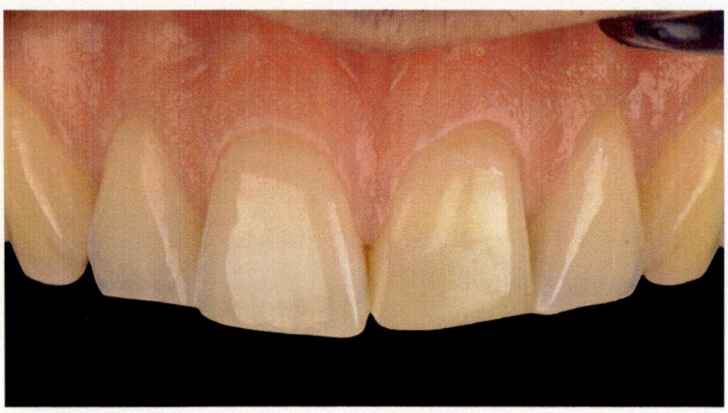

Figure 1 Initial situation of the upper jaw: tooth 21 has an old restoration which requires replacement.

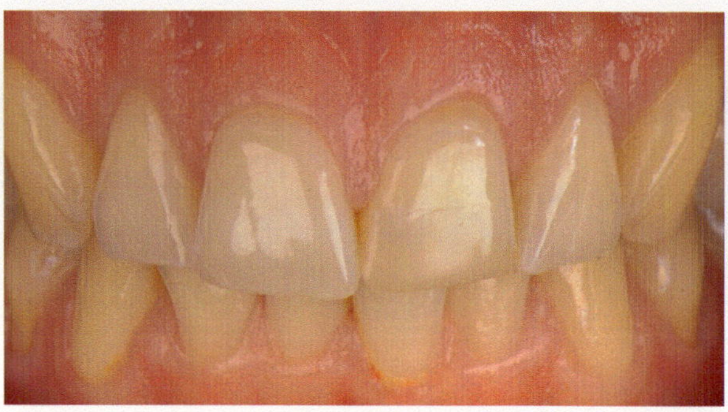

Figure 2 Inital situation in relation to the lower jaw.

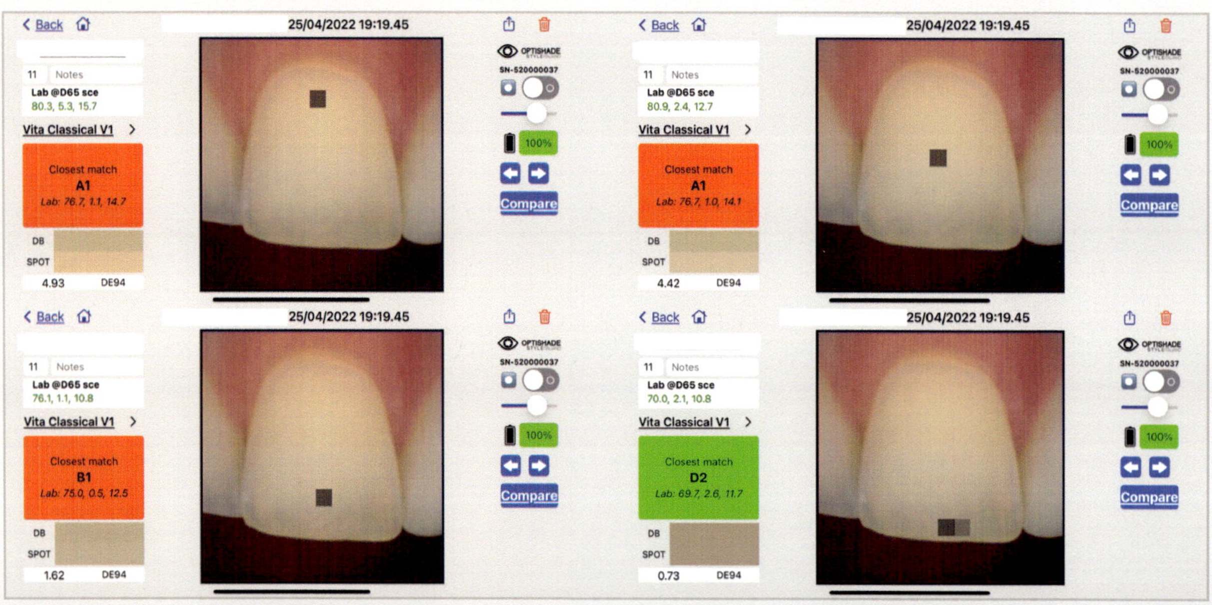

Figure 3 The Optishade measurements of the tooth show a range of different shades between A1, B1 and D2. The red square indicates a clear difference with the proposed Vita shade tab. The green square shows a close match. Using this shade mapping, the recipe can be chosen.

To facilitate the shaping of the restoration, a palatal putty is made on a direct or indirect wax-up of the tooth before the start of the treatment. In this case, however, neither were done. Instead, a palatal putty was taken of the present situation and the putty was then adjusted to increase the length and adjust the shape of tooth 21. This palatal reference facilitates future layering. When playing with the contrast of the initial picture (4), a translucent zone can be observed in the incisal quarter of the tooth, marked with the dotted line. This can also be recreated in the restoration.

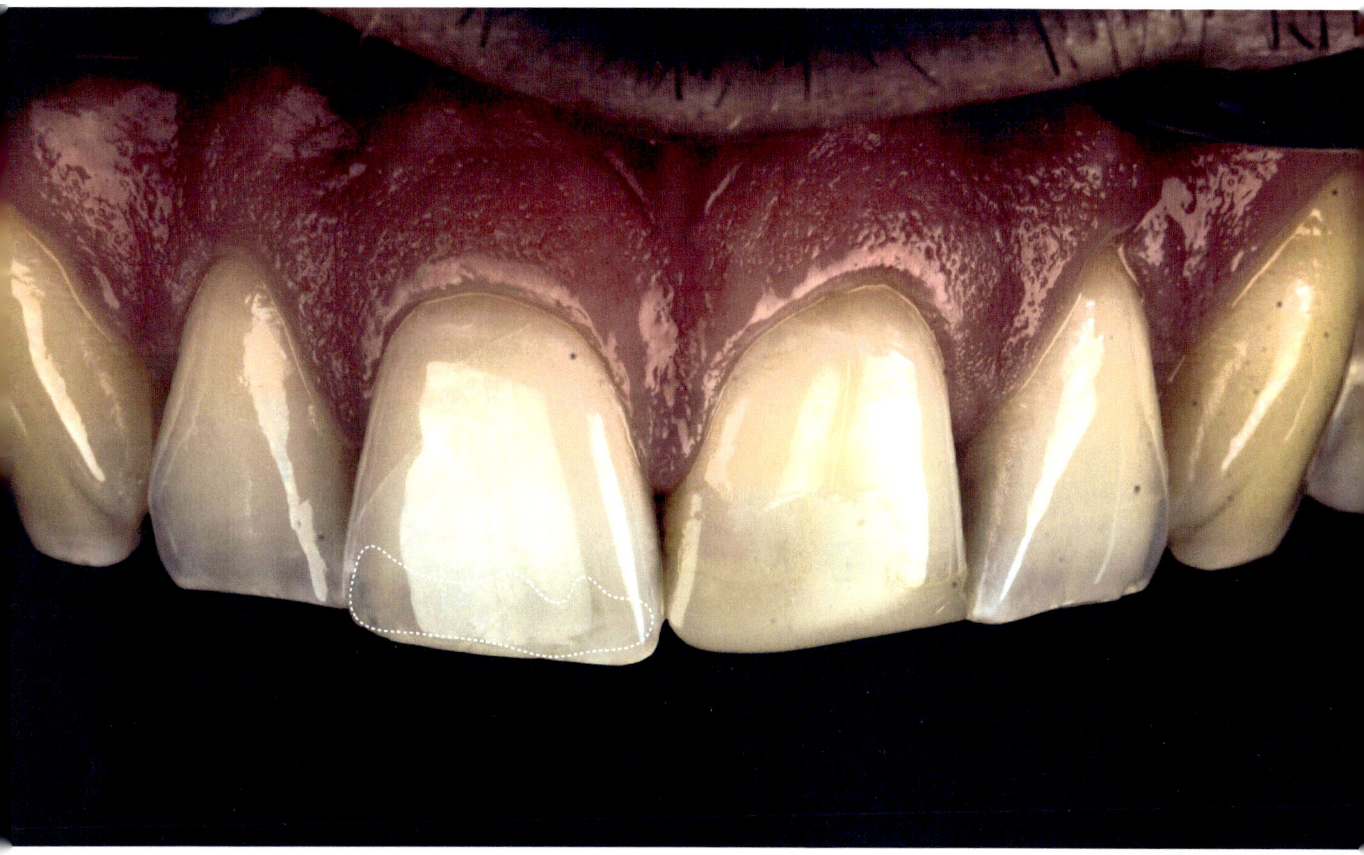

Figure 4 Altered image of figure 1, to reveal intrinsic anatomy of the teeth. The dotted line on tooth 11 shows a more translucent zone which can be replicated in the new restoration.

After anesthesia and rubber dam placement, using a slow speed ceramic round bur, the tooth-composite border is identified (5). This technique allows to faster remove the remainder of the more incisal composite. The entire incisal third of the tooth was previously lost and now needs to be replaced with a new restoration (6, 7). To make sure that the new restoration blends in nicely with the remainder of the tooth, an adequate bevel was made. Figure 8 (8) shows the mesial view of tooth 21 with the design of the previous bevel. When beveling anterior teeth, the bevel should be invasive enough to allow a gradient between the newly added restoration and the tooth, in order to make the transition invisible to the human eye. The old bevel was long and shallow, resulting in more visible finish line (if microhybrid composite was

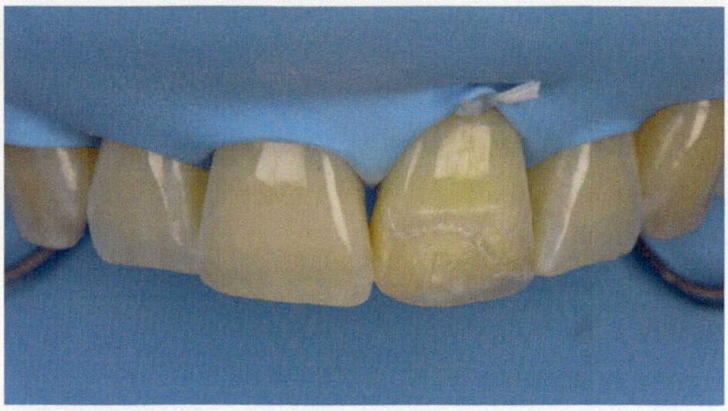

Figure 5 Isolated view of the upper anterior jaw. A floss ligature is placed to increase the view and workspace on tooth 21. The margin of the old restoration is identified with a round ceramic, slow speed bur.

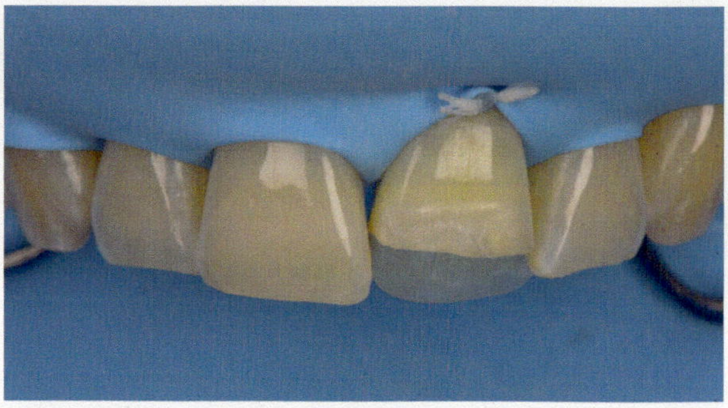

Figure 6 Overlap of the old restoration and the remaining tooth structure.

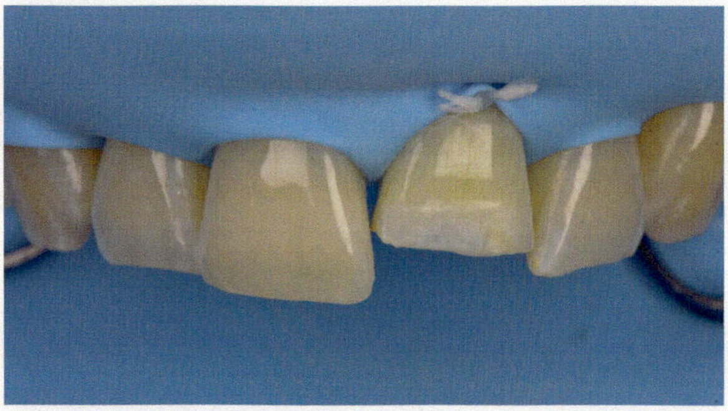

Figure 7 Tooth 21 after removing the old restoration.

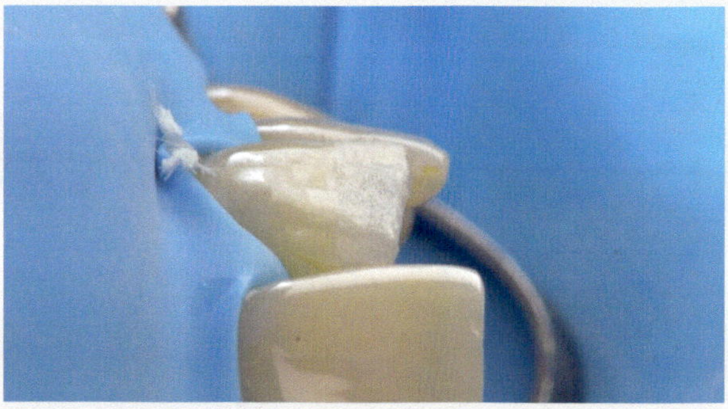

Figure 8 The mesial view of tooth 21 showing the old bevel and preparation.

used) and a possibility to distinguish the cut-off line. A rounded infinite bevel was prepared to ensure a smooth transition; in 📷 9 all steps to create such a bevel are described. This bevel will effectively mask the cut-off point and, in combination with a nano-hybrid composite, the finish line should become invisible. A fine diamond bur can be used to create the two first bevels of 45 and 20 degrees. The rounding is easily done with a coarse diamond finishing disc, which will also polish the beveled enamel, creating a smooth surface to bond to, as can be observed in the last picture. The smooth enamel and rounded shape can be observed in the buccal and incisal views of the bevel (📷 10). Notice the tooth is endodontically treated, but no avital bleaching was done beforehand.

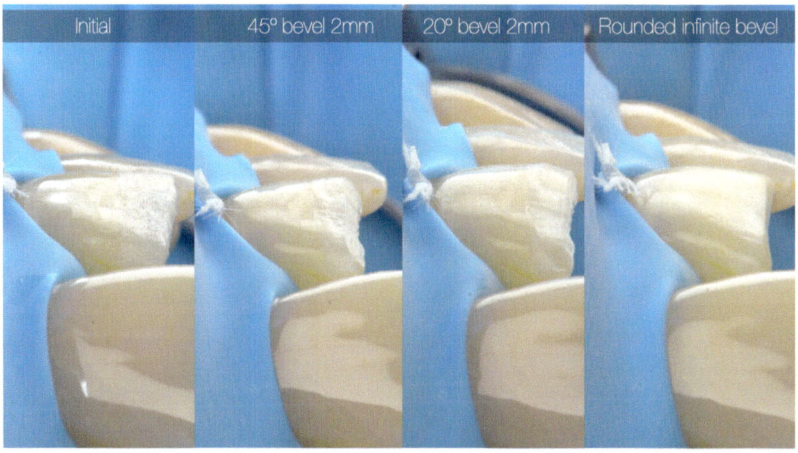

Figure 9 Mesial view of tooth 21 for each step of the new bevelling procedure. After having cleared all old restoration remnants, a first bevel of about 1 mm wide under a 45 degree angle is cut. Censequently a 20 degree bevel is cut until a width of about 2 mm is reached. To finalized all bevels are connected and edges are rounded using a coarse finishing disc.

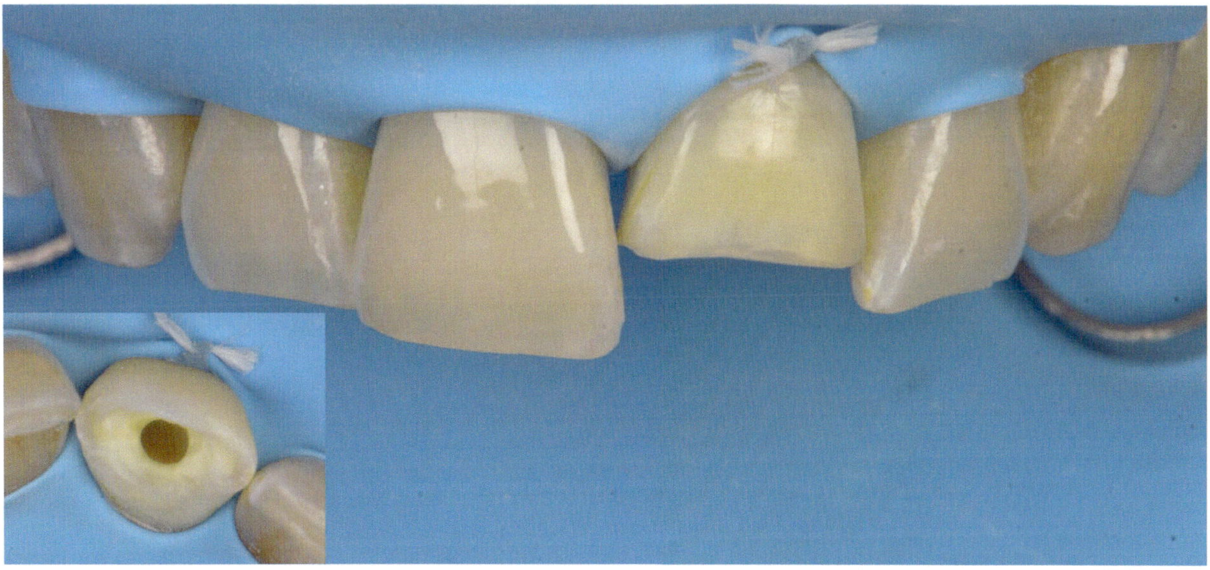

Figure 10 Buccal and incisal view of the bevelled tooth 21.

Two posterior matrices (Lumicontrast, Polydentia, Switzerland) are inserted interproximal with the outside towards the tooth that needs to be treated (📷 11). This way the neighboring teeth are protected during etching and adhesive application procedures. The universal adhesive was applied after selective enamel etching by gently rubbing for 20 seconds. After soft air blowing, the adhesive was light cured for 20 seconds. On the dentin a thin layer of flowable composite was applied as a resin coat and light cured for 10 seconds. This is to protect the hybrid layer from inherent shrinkage stress occurring after placing the following layers of packable composite. It also creates a flowing surface without imperfections from burs or decay. This will prevent air bubble inclusion when adding the next layers.

The putty is fitted (📷 12), and the palatal margin can be marked with a sharp instrument so a clear mark is visible to know where the composite has to be placed. See how the

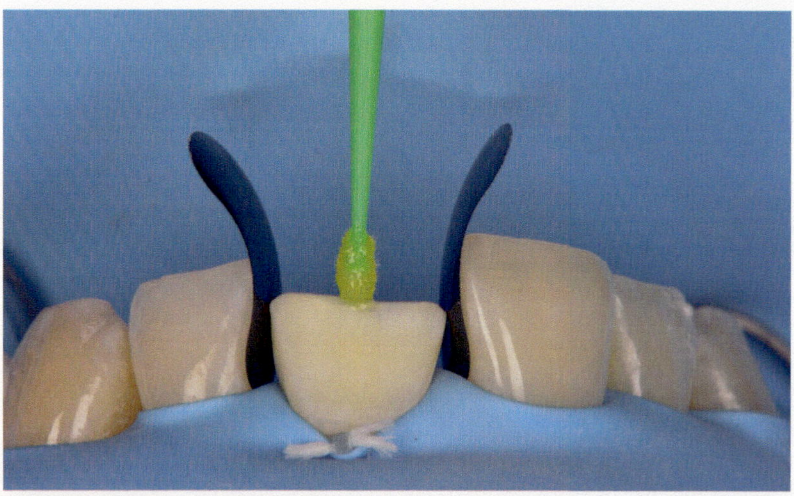

Figure 11 Buccal view of the sandblasted and selectively enamel etched tooth 21. Lumicontrast matrices in "protection mode" and application of the self etch adhesive.

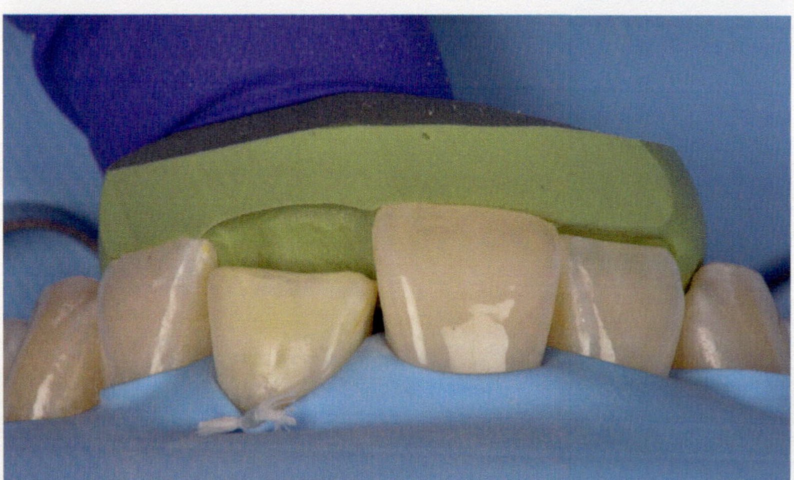

Figure 12 Placement of the palatal putty index, light pressure is needed to keep it in place.

index is shaped to be symmetrical to the contralateral central incisor. This putty index is used to create the "palatal shell". A thin layer of composite will represent the first layer of the restoration and will provide support for the subsequent layers. In the recipe a thick base layer of high value dentin composite was chosen, this means the initial thickness of the palatal shell is of less importance (13) . Only in the incisal aspect there needs to be sufficient room to layer the second layer of composite and some characterisation. It is important to place the palatal shell composite a little bit over (about 1mm) the previously applied mark to ensure adequate fit to the palatal wall and to reduce the risk of air bubbles, voids, and loosening of the palatal shell consequently.

The remainder of the dentin mass is applied and space is left in the incisal quarter for characterization. Also, space is left interproximally for the enamel layering (14). A simple form is chosen as in the neighboring tooth no extreme mamelons were differentiated

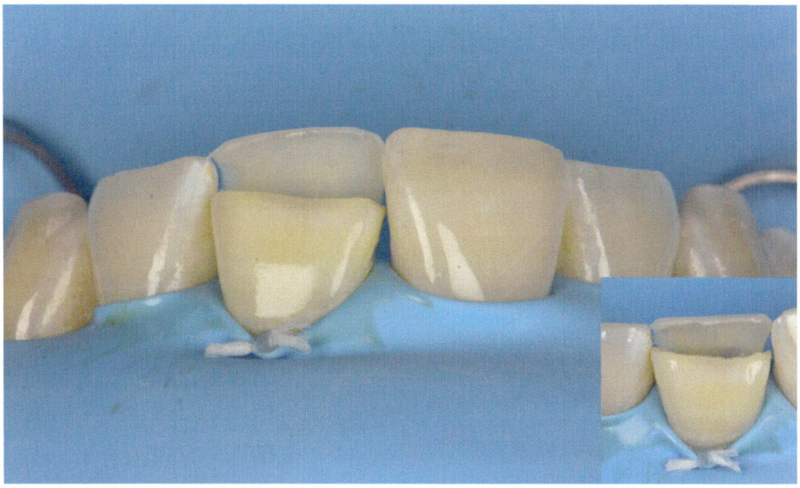

Figure 13 The palatal shell from a buccal and bucco-incisal view.

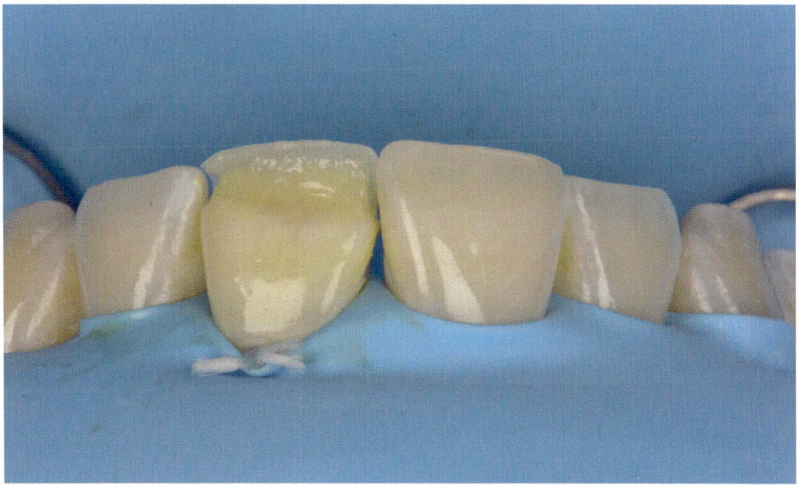

Figure 14 Placement of the dentin layer, no difficult mamelon pattern was chosen.

followed by placement of translucent effect composite for small characterization of the previously observed translucent incisal space. Also, the interproximal walls were built up in the more translucent shade (📷 15). The buccal layer is now easy to apply using the LM Arte Solo Anterior instrument (LM, Finland). The spatula is very versatile and facilitates pasting the composite in place in a homogeneous layer. Because of the large surface area that can be used, the finishing is facilitated by the low number of irregularities in the previous layers and bevel (📷 16).

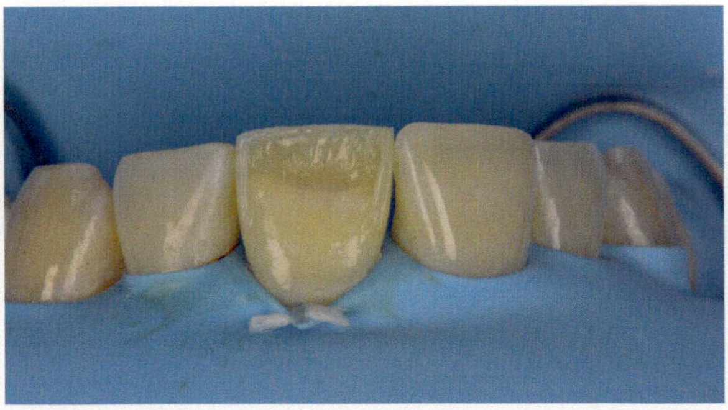

Figure 15 Interproximal walls are build.

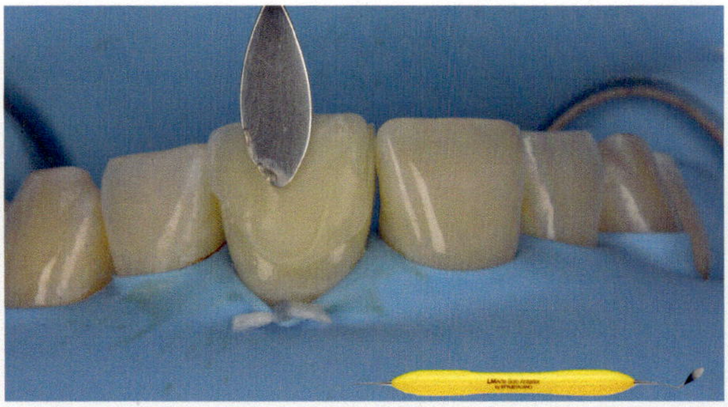

Figure 16 Placement of the final buccal layer with the LM Solo Anterior instrument.

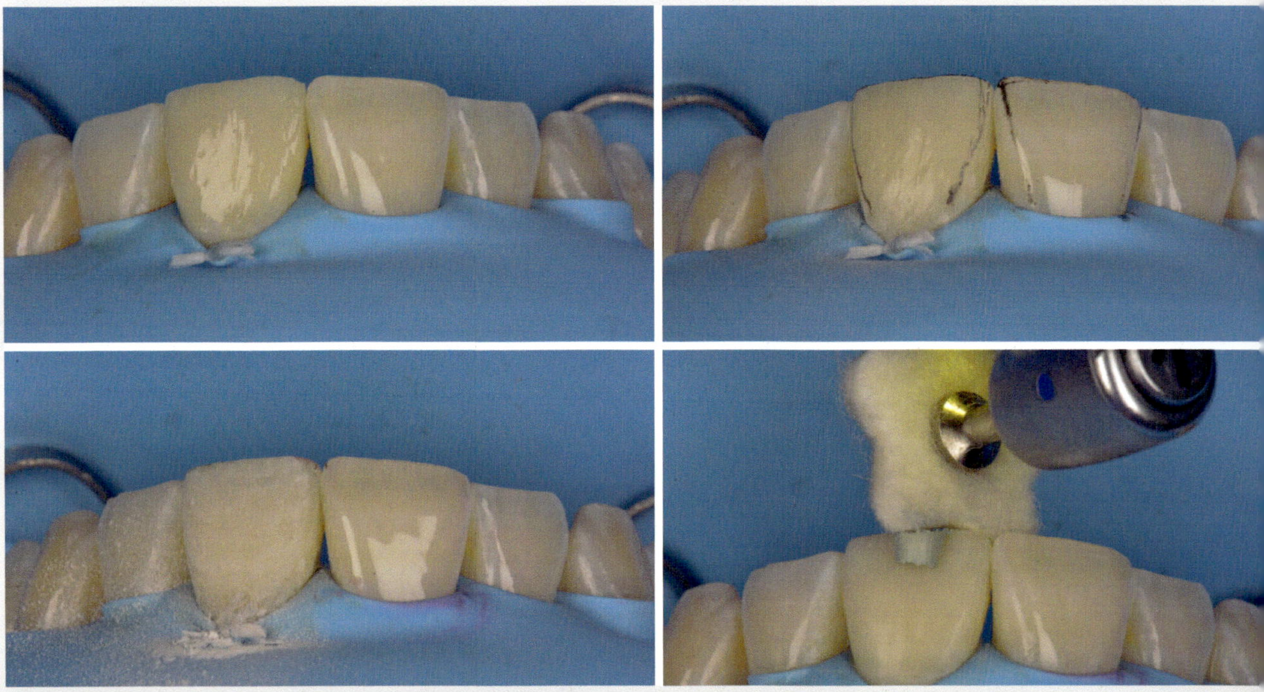

Figure 17 After application of the last layer, a slight over contour can be noticed. The outlines are marked with pencil and are finished with slow rotating burs and discs. Finally, application of the Lucida paste and polishing with the Lucida star-shaped felt wheel are performed.

The finishing and polishing steps (📷 17) were done following the Shape technique by StyleItaliano[5], which provides a final surface texture and gloss that mimics the neighboring tooth as closely as possible (📷 18). After removing the rubber dam, the surface texture can be re-examined under normal light circumstances and adjusted where needed; in this case nothing was changed (📷 19, 20).

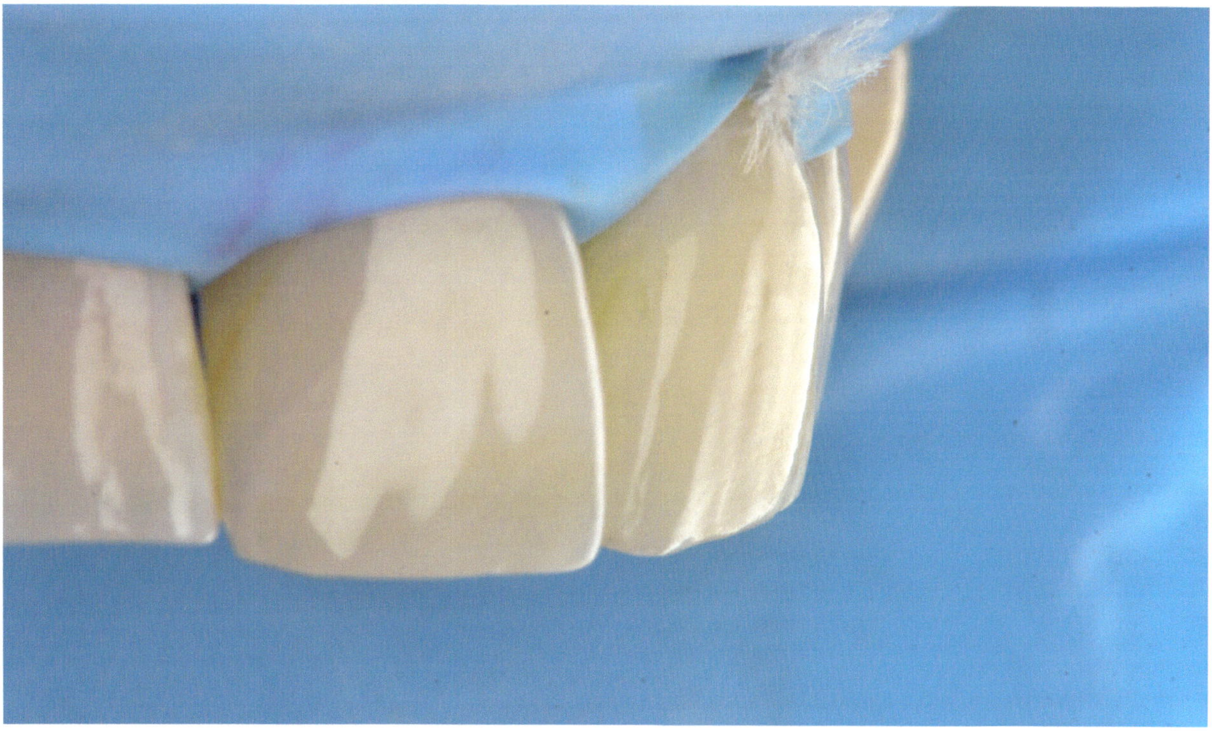

Figure 18 Side view with lighting to show the secondary anatomy enhanced by the luster.

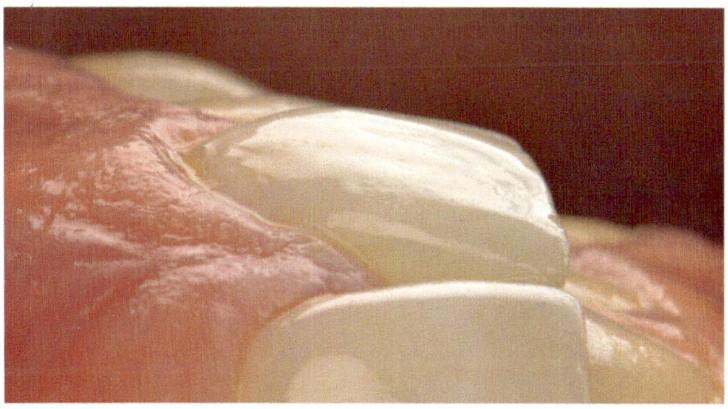

Figure 19 Immediate side view of tooth 21 after rubberdam removal.

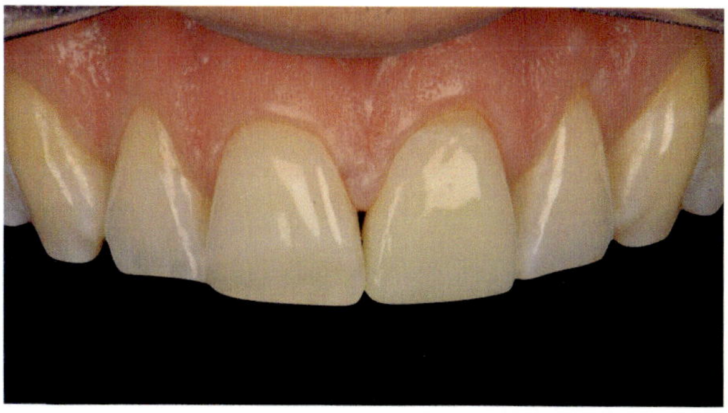

Figure 20 Immediate result, notice the dehydration of the teeth in general.

The result 2 weeks after placement of the restoration, visible in 21 shows a nice symmetry between both central incisors. Furthermore, the shade matching is satisfactory to the naked eye. Using the "compare" function in the Optishade app, two weeks after placement, the measurements are set side by side **(22)**. As can be observed, a score of 1.77 was achieved following the recipe as prescribed. An untrained person will not be able to see the difference below a Delta E value of 3. While a Delta E <1 is visually imperceptible **(23, 24)**, a professional could see a slight difference when Delta E is between 1 and 2.

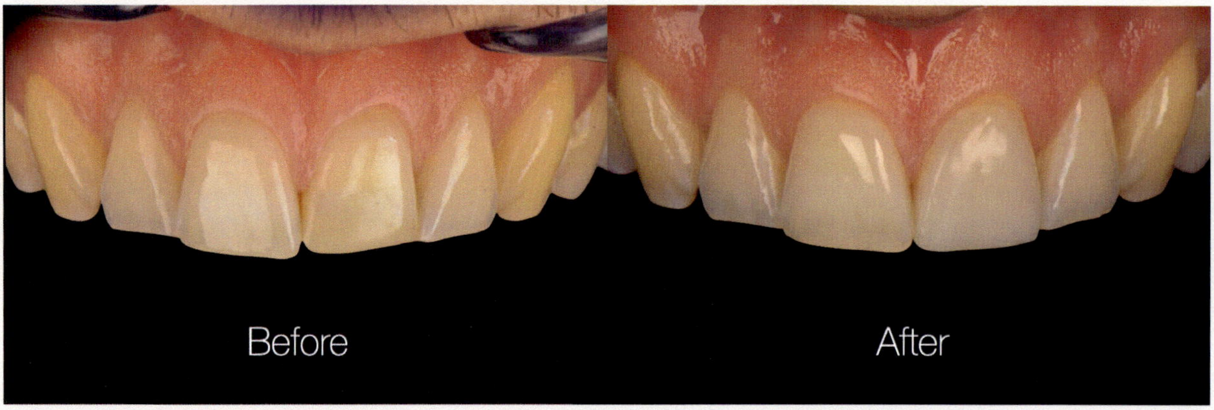

Figure 21 The before and after two weeks picture showing the result of the treatment.

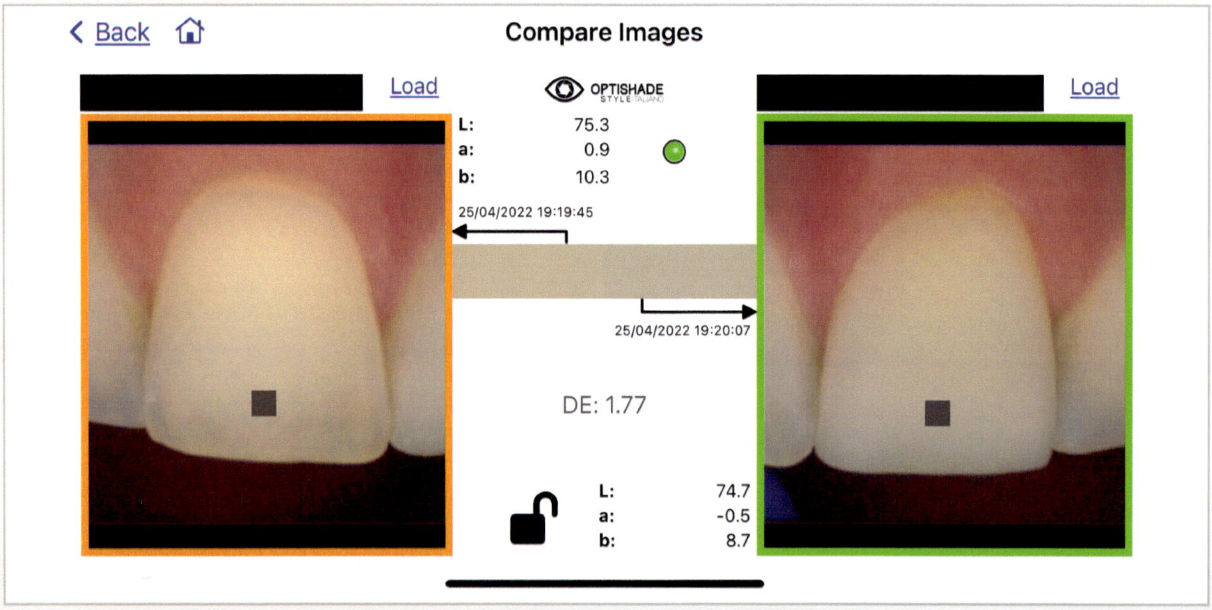

Figure 22 Optishade measurements comparing the tooth 11 and tooth 21 shades the Delta E is 1.77.

In another case, multiple teeth had to be restored after having used clear aligners, using the same workflow (12, 11, 21, 22) (25). A direct mock-up was performed to test the length of the teeth and the chosen shades (26). This was also used to create a palatal putty. The old restoration on tooth 21 was removed and enamel was treated for adhesion (27). On 28 the palatal shell is in place as well as the dentin layer and effects. A roll of white opaque composite is used to create the halo effect on the incisal edge. After final finishing and polishing, the luster is achieved through usage of the Diashine Lucida polishing system (29).

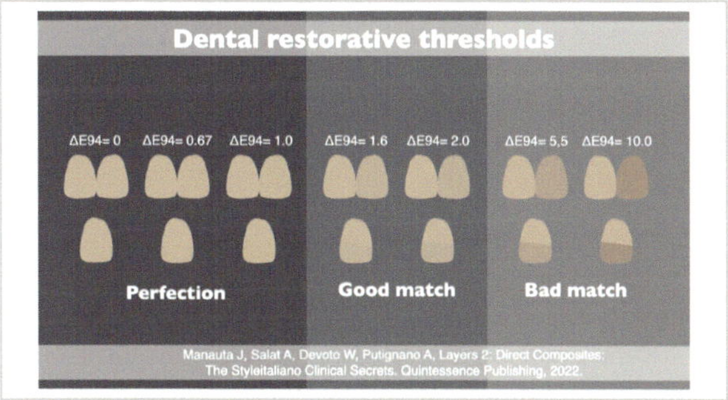

Figure 23 Restorative thresholds visualized with pictograms.

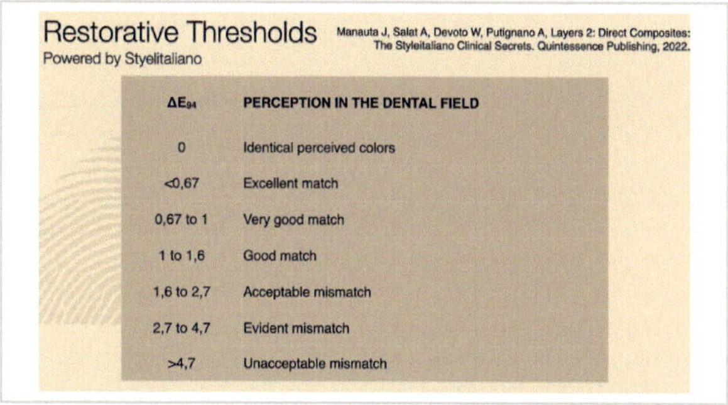

Restorative Thresholds
Powered by Styelitaliano

Manauta J, Salat A, Devoto W, Putignano A, Layers 2: Direct Composites: The Styleitaliano Clinical Secrets. Quintessence Publishing, 2022.

ΔE_{94}	PERCEPTION IN THE DENTAL FIELD
0	Identical perceived colors
<0,67	Excellent match
0,67 to 1	Very good match
1 to 1,6	Good match
1,6 to 2,7	Acceptable mismatch
2,7 to 4,7	Evident mismatch
>4,7	Unacceptable mismatch

Figure 24 Restorative thresholds explained in numbers.

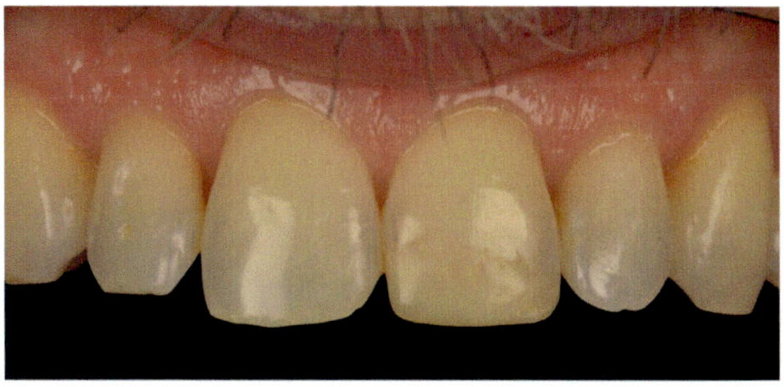

Figure 25 Initial situation of case 2, the patient wanted to replace the restoration on tooth 21 and enhance the shape of the remaining incisors.

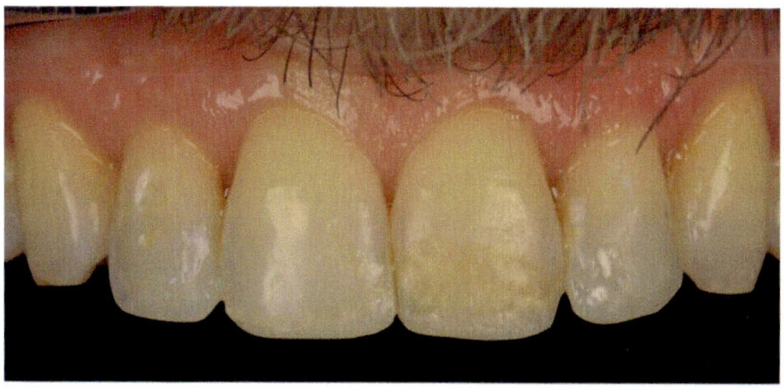

Figure 26 A quick mock up to test shape and shade were done and validated by the patient.

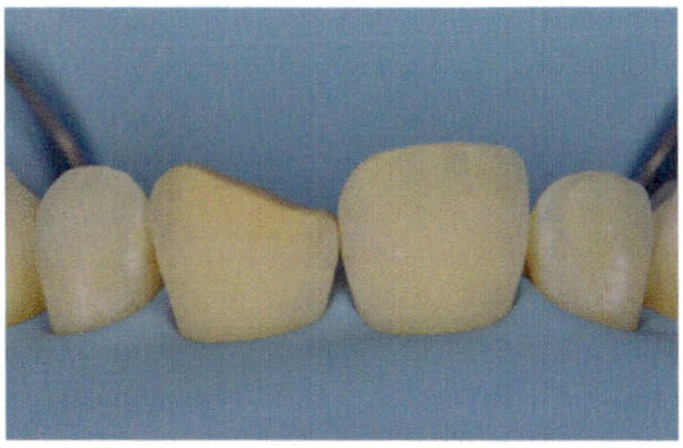

Figure 27 Preparation of all teeth was done by removing the old restorations, rounding sharp edges and air abraiding all surfaces.

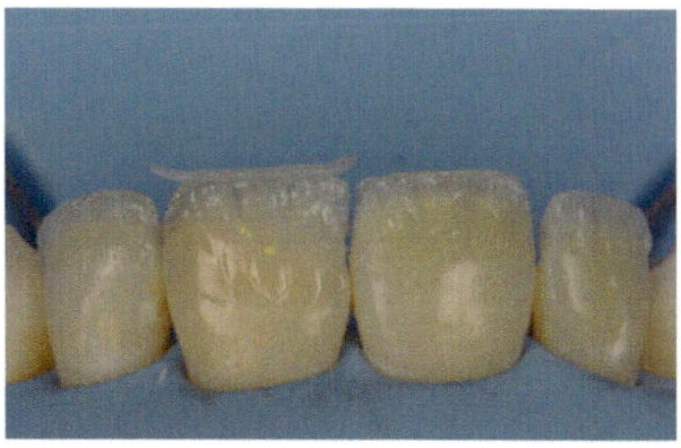

Figure 28 The build-up phase of the restorations.

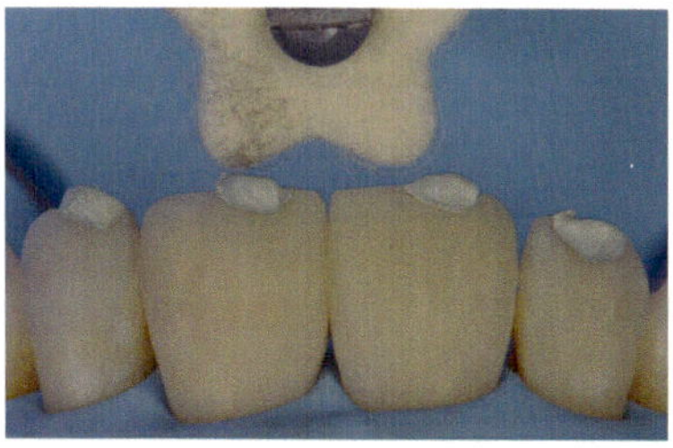

Figure 29 Final polishing step with the Lucida system.

The polished surface reflects nicely the created secondary and tertiary anatomy (30, 31, 32). Upon three weeks the final shade matching can be appreciated, which is also visible on the Optishade measurements (33, 34, 35, 36).

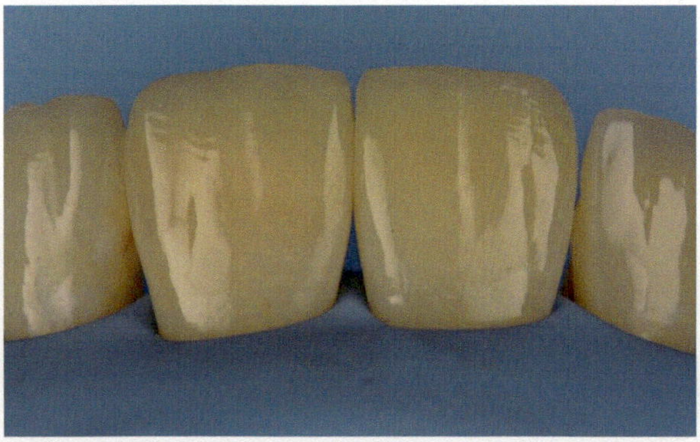

Figure 30 Final polishing revealing the final shape and texture of the restorations.

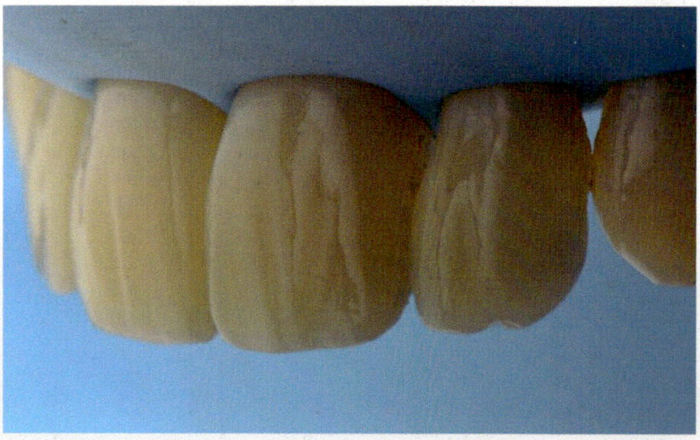

Figure 31 Side view of the restorations extra time was spent creating a natural young secondary and tertiary anatomy.

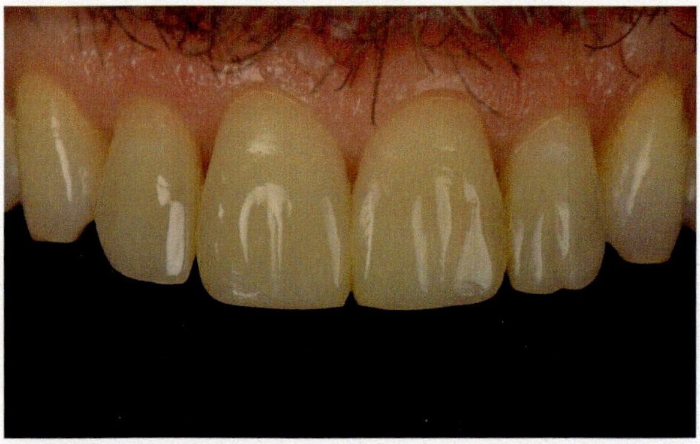

Figure 32 Integration of the restorations 2 weeks after placement.

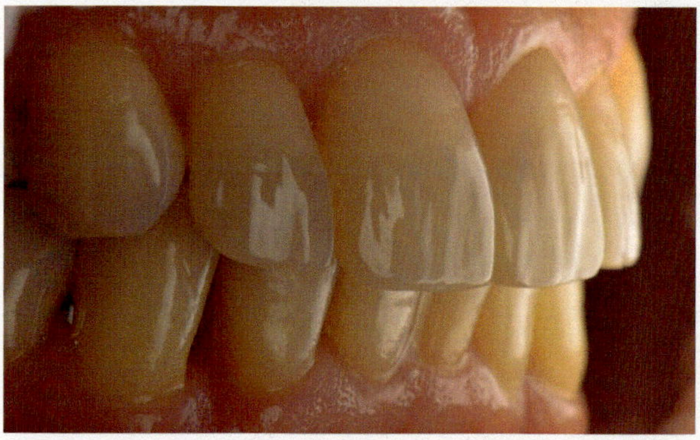

Figure 33 Side view of the restorations in relation to the lower jaw, 3 weeks post-op.

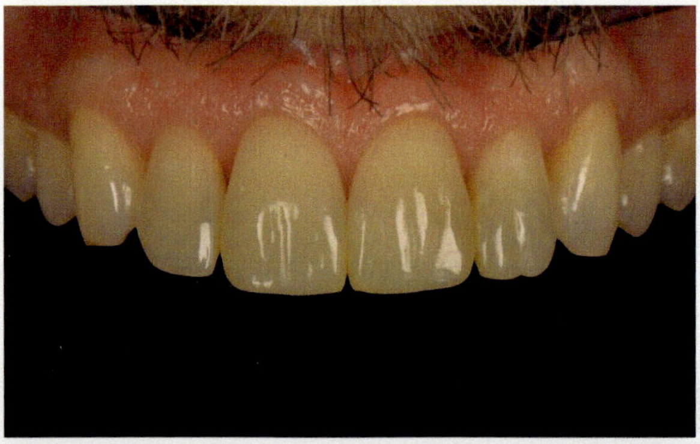

Figure 34 Final view, 3 weeks post-op.

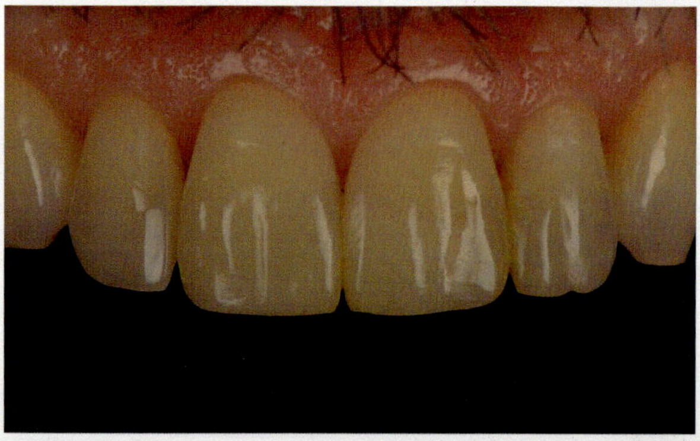

Figure 35 Close-up view of the post-op result.

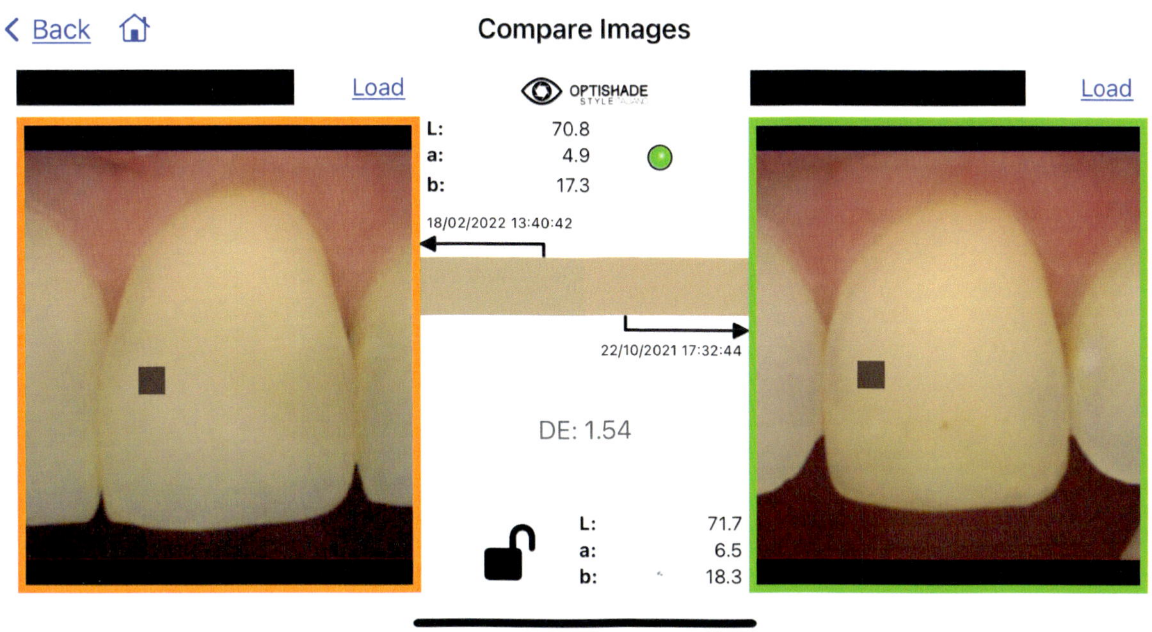

Figure 36 Optishade measurement showing the match of the restoration with the original tooth shade.

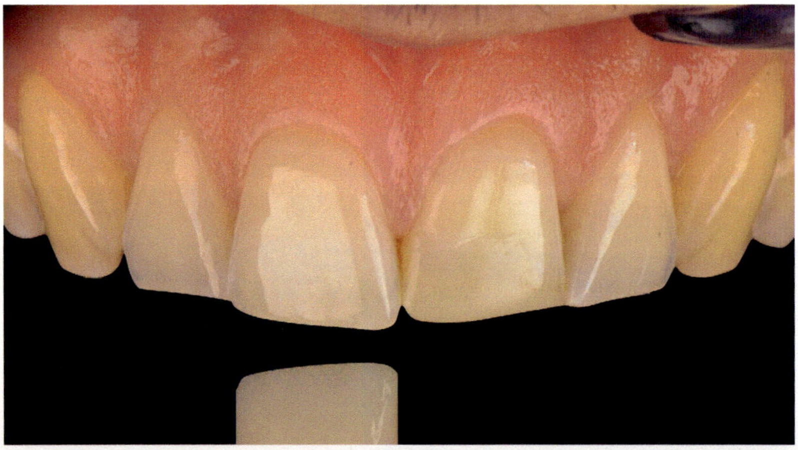

Figure 37 A direct self made shade guide can be used to verify the composite recipe.

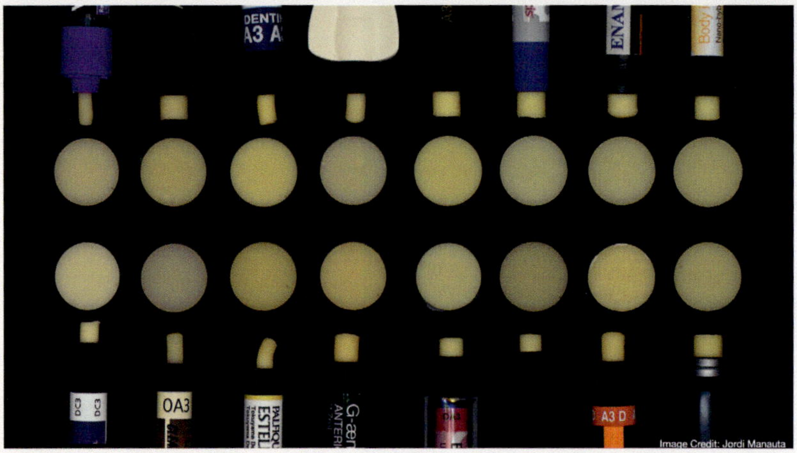

Figure 38 A3 composites samples form different brands.

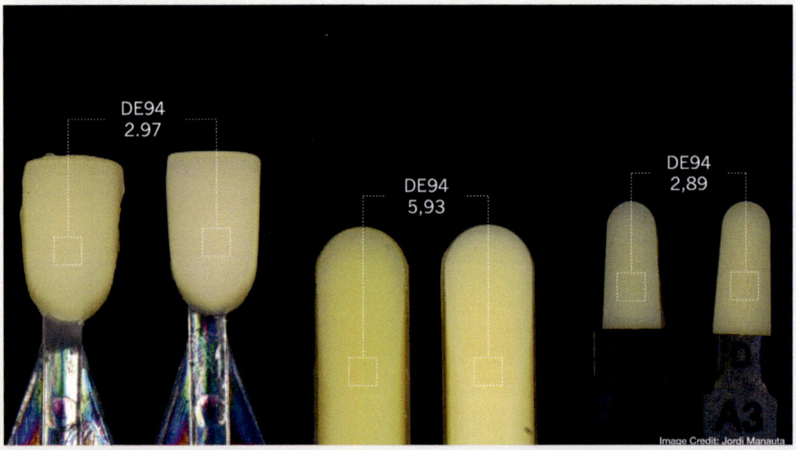

Figure 39 Delta E differences between different brand A3 shades.

CONCLUSIONS

Using this shade-mapping, it is easier to understand what shades are mixed throughout the tooth. An estimation of the resulting Delta E is also projected, which reflects the predictability of the given shade. It could be interesting to know that an A1 shade might be the closest shade to the tooth, but will still differ significantly to be seen by the naked eye (Delta E>1). But by using a mixture of different shades/translucencies/thicknesses, the dentist will be able to achieve a color match closer to the real shade. By doing a direct mock-up or creating a personalized shade guide based on a self-made recipe, we can verify the color instantly as seen in **37**. This can also be seen in **38, 39** where A3 shades of numerous different composite systems were compared to one another. Also, the shade guides themselves are not consistent, which makes it even more complex[3]. Every tooth has another shade, translucency, and dimension, which all influence how we should layer our different shades and translucencies.

BIBLIOGRAPHY

1. Ismail EH, Dawson DV, Maia RR, et al. A novel sample design for determining color compatibility between layered resin composite and vita shade guides. *Journal of Esthetic and Restorative Dentistry: official publication of the American Academy of Esthetic Dentistry*. 2020;32(1):34-42.
2. Browning WD, Contreras-Bulnes R, Brackett MG, Brackett WW. Color differences: polymerized composite and corresponding Vitapan Classical Shade Tab. *Journal of Dentistry*. 2009;37 Suppl 1:e34-9.
3. King KA, deRijk WG. Variations of L*a*b* values among Vitapan Classical Shade Guides. *Journal of Prosthodontics: official journal of the American College of Prosthodontists*. 2007;16(5):352-26.
4. Manauta J & Salat A. *Layers: An Atlas of Composite Resin Stratification*. Quintessence Pub. 2012; pp. 58-67.
5. Manauta J, Salat A, Devoto W, Putignano A. *Layers 2: Direct Composites: The StyleItaliano Clinical Secrets*. Quintessence Pub. 2022.

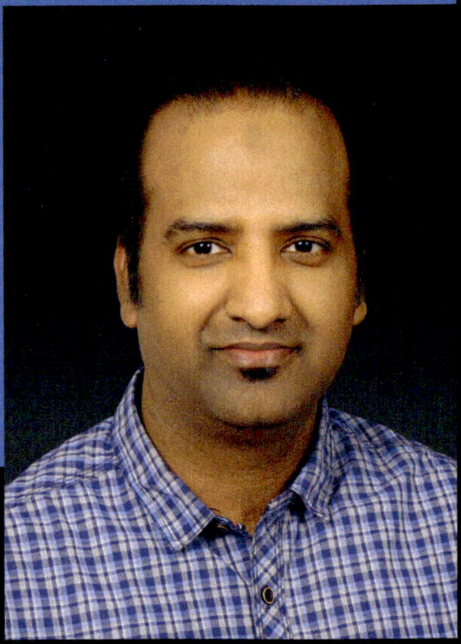

ZUHAIR ARIF

Pakistan

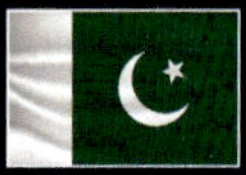

Dr Zuhair Arif obtained his degree in Dental Medicine from University Of Health Sciences of Lahore (Pakistan), in 2008.
In 2016 he completed his fellowship in Operative Dentistry from College of Physicians and Surgeons (Karachi, Pakistan). He was appointed Assistant Professor at the Department of Operative Dentistry of Akhtar Saeed Medical and Dental College, Lahore, and he recently started his career as Consultant of Restorative Dentistry in Saudi Arabia.
Dr Zuhair Arif has been lecturing in seminars, giving hands-on courses, and performing live case demonstrations on esthetic dentistry and composite applications. He has been working with StyleItaliano since 2018 and he has also contributed to *Layers 2* (Quintessence pub.), a book of StyleItaliano techniques.
Dr Zuhair Arif's focus is now to be at fore front of Esthetic Dentistry and Dental Photography.

TAKING A SHORTCUT IN THE MASTERING OF POSTERIOR COMPOSITE MODELING

Since their introduction in the early 1970s, dental composite resins have become a routine for anterior and posterior restorations. Their ability to be adhesively placed allows for highly conservative and non-invasive preparations, and they are capable of reinforcing the remaining parts of tooth structure, giving these restorative materials a definite advantage over silver amalgam.

It is well known among clinicians that, even if there are no unequivocal data, all methods of placing composite resin in a cavity aim to increase the free surface of the material and to decrease the configuration factor. This is independent from the horizontal, vertical, or oblique layering technique applied.

The choice of layering is mandatory when the final cavity design is deeper than 2 mm.

The excellent optical and structural features of modern composite resin materials, allow us to provide an esthetic appearance to something that must be, first of all, functionally correct. In order to provide a correct shape and function, a reliable modeling technique will give us higher quality restoration.

DISCUSSION AND CLINICAL CASE

Advantages of Modeling

- Less finishing time
- Less occlusion corrections
- Better sealing
- Less stress

At the beginning of my profession, I had no knowledge of tooth morphology or the various modeling procedures, and some of the early cases and exercises I published at the beginning of the article are some of my least successful one.

In order to improve my dental skills, I began to follow the StyleItaliano Group. I read through their 2012 book, *Layers*, published by Quintessence pub., I followed their clinical tips and went through their cases. The procedures for anterior and posterior restorations were all explained in this book, along with layering techniques of posterior teeth including "Pizza Technique" and the "Espresso Posterior Technique".

Thus, in brief, layering is necessary: first, to compensate for the intrinsic limits resulting from the chemistry of composite materials, and second, but no less importantly, because there is not and there will never be function without morphology, regardless of the esthetic.

I was practicing routine dentistry, using a low-resolution camera, not paying attention to the anatomy of the tooth, and always thinking that my work was fine. In reality, I was in a fool's paradise; just consider the outcomes if I had no idea about tooth anatomy and tried to copy it, what would happen? And if I had captured details with a low-resolution camera without documenting my cases, how could I have believed that my dentistry was error-free? I would have continued to make the same mistakes, fooling myself into believing that I was competent. However, after reading StyleItaliano's articles, I realized that beautiful work does not come naturally; it requires practice, photographic skills, and perfect documentation, which you should display to others in order to identify your mistakes. I vividly remember the time I looked at my clinical case using a DSLR camera and was disappointed by the low quality of restoration. Then I began my exercises, focusing on my photography and case documentation skills, and after four years I could really tell a difference.

Benefits of Extraoral Exercises

- Mistakes and unseen details in exercises are amplified in the real clinical cases.
- Keeping the samples allows the operator to see mistakes.

Examples of Beginner Exercises

Exercise 1

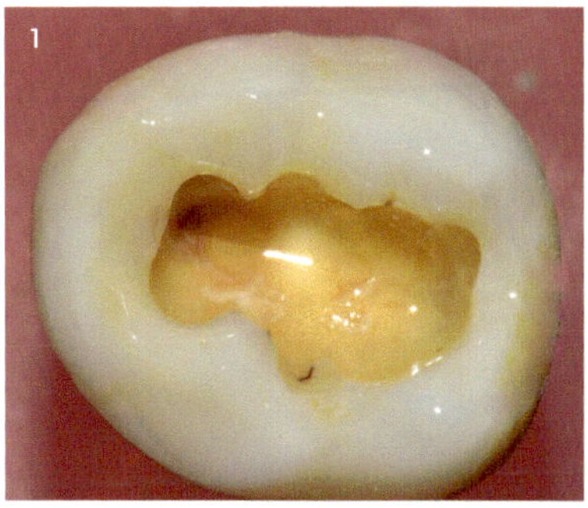

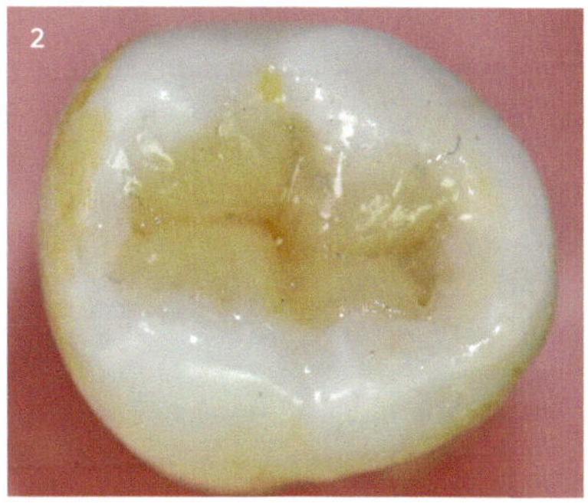

Figure 1 The initial picture of tooth 36 shows that cavity preparation was done poorly.

Figure 2 Post-operative picture showing wrong anatomy of mandibular first molar and poor details.

Exercise 2

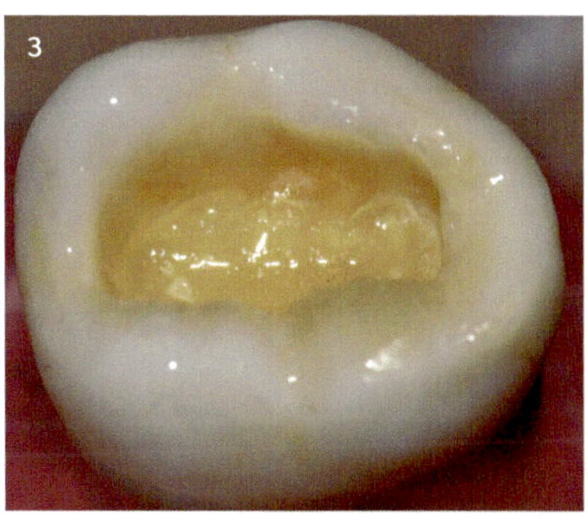

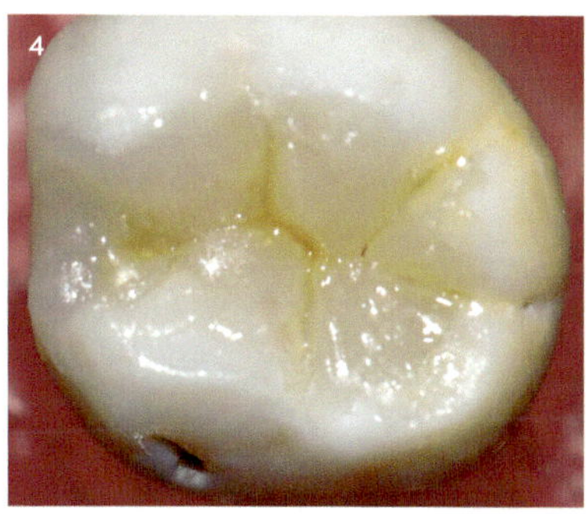

Figure 3 Initial situation of cavity with poor cavity preparation.

Figure 4 Final image.

Exercise 3

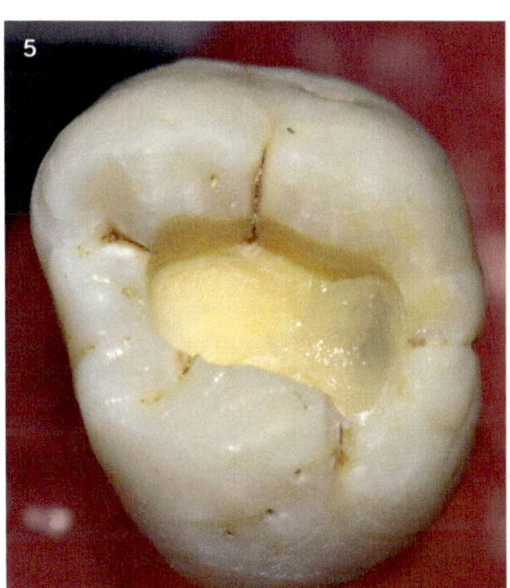

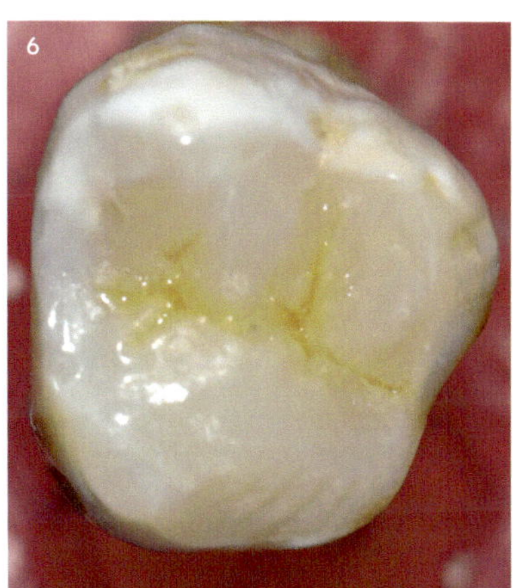

Figure 5 Initial situation of cavity.

Figure 6 Final image.

Clinical Case 1

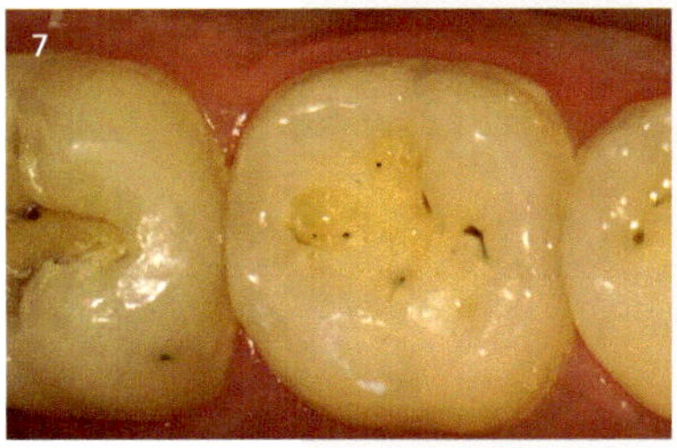

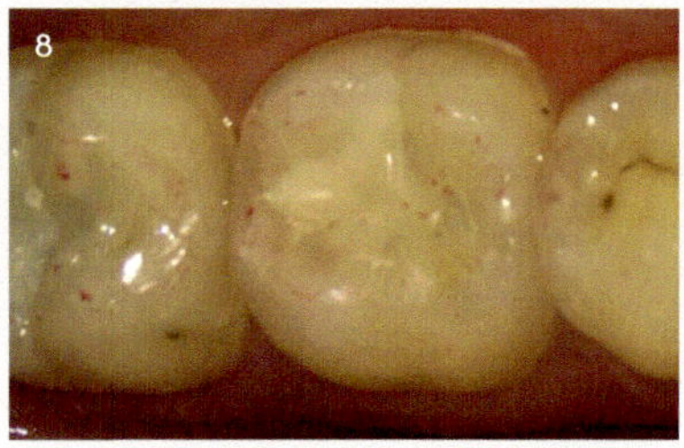

Figure 7 An old case done in 2018.

Figure 8 Final picture showing poor adaptation of composite.

"YOUR LIFE DOES NOT GET BETTER BY CHANCE, IT GETS BETTER BY CHANGE" – JIM ROHAN –

After completing many exercises, wasting a lot of materials, and using every available instrument, I came to the conclusion that using smart materials and specialized instruments is just as important as studying and reading literature. As a result, I started using LM Arte composite instruments, as well as purchasing my DSLR camera, and I soon began to see positive results and bigger steps in my evolution.

Thanks to their wonderful book, *Layers*, by StyleItaliano where I learned about the Pizza Technique, my results were amazing and I started to put this technique into practice in my extra-oral exercises and later in my clinical cases. I love pizza (successive cusp technique) and never imagined that one day I could build teeth sections that look like pizza slices. After mastering it, I moved on to exploring other techniques, among which is the Espresso Technique.

The Pizza Technique

The successive cusp builds up were described in 1996 by Liebenbergh. Even this technique provides amazing clinical outcomes, it's more time-consuming but less affected by contraction. Pizza technique is a modification of the incremental layering technique. This technique is done by applying one layer to each tooth cusp. Each of these layers when formed resembles slices of pizza. The procedure starts with a simple cusp then adds another cusp to obtain a shape that is more in accordance with natural anatomy.

Exercise 4

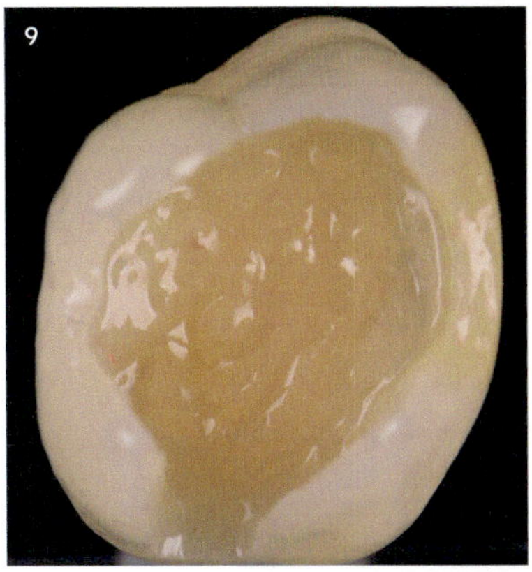

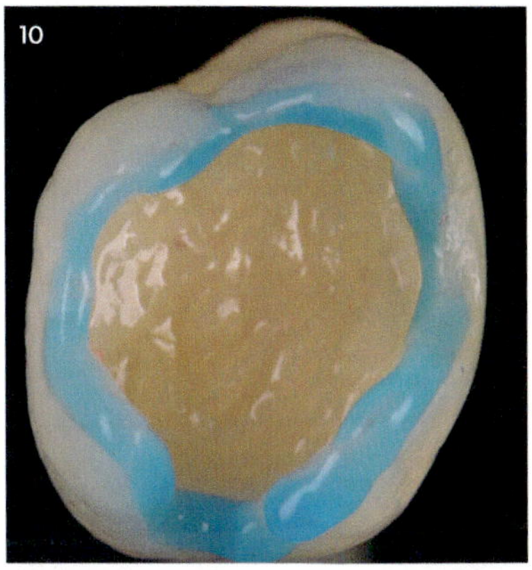

Figure 9 Initial image of cavity.

Figure 10 Selective etching of the enamel with 37 percent orthophosphoric acid and universal adhesive applied.

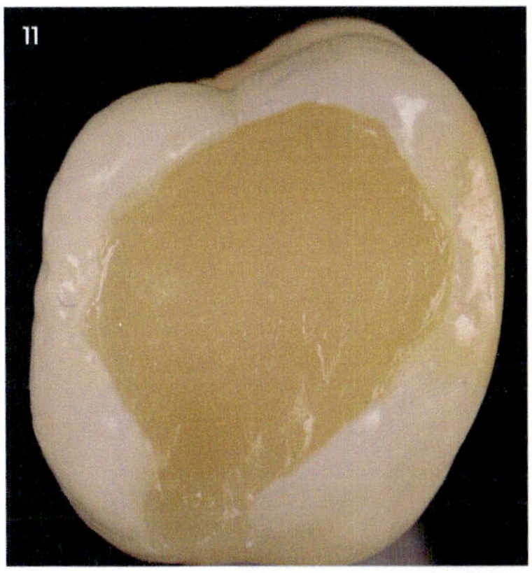

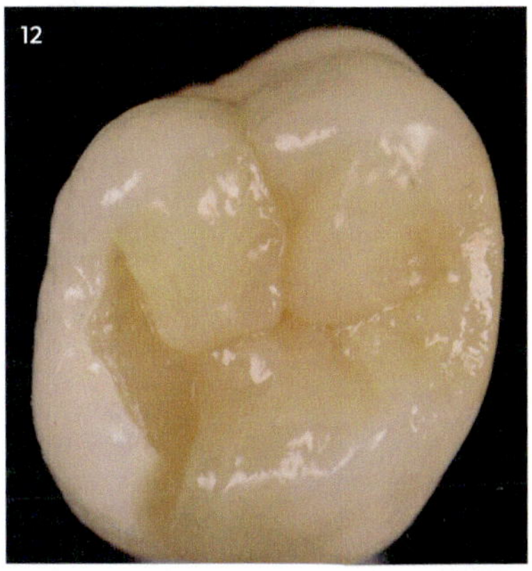

Figure 11 The bulk material was then placed in just one increment. The single increment offered by the features of bulk material was an advantage in this case, as a 4-5 mm layer could be placed at once.

Figure 12 Tooth modeling with Pizza Technique.

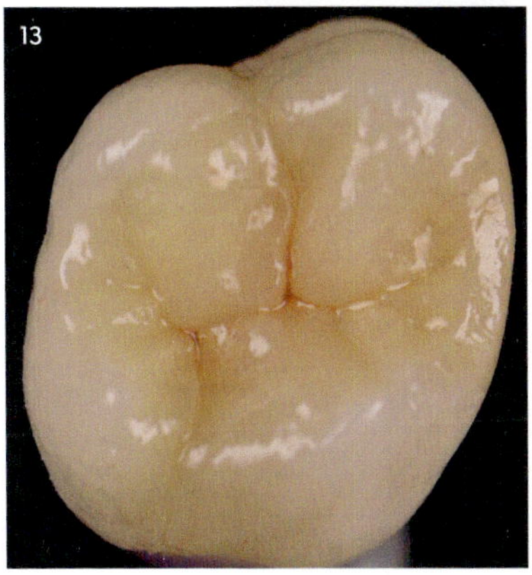

Figure 13 Final image after finishing and polishing with Lucida.

Side-by-Side Cavities

The satisfactory direct composite restoration of a proximal surface in class-11 cavities requires fulfillment of several criteria, including attainment of an anatomically correct contour and tight contact area, adequate marginal adaptation, and accurate marginal ring placement. Matrices are need to be placed simultaneously, with the advantages of time saving and of preventing contamination of neighboring cavities during treatment.

Clinical Case 2 (Pizza Technique)

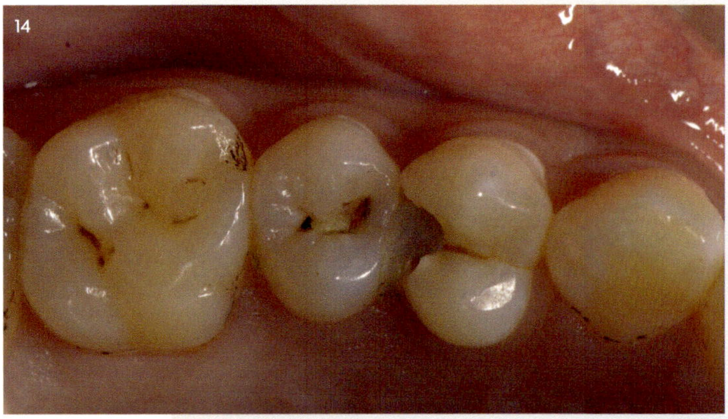

Figure 14 This is an image of left upper quadrant of a 30-years old patient.

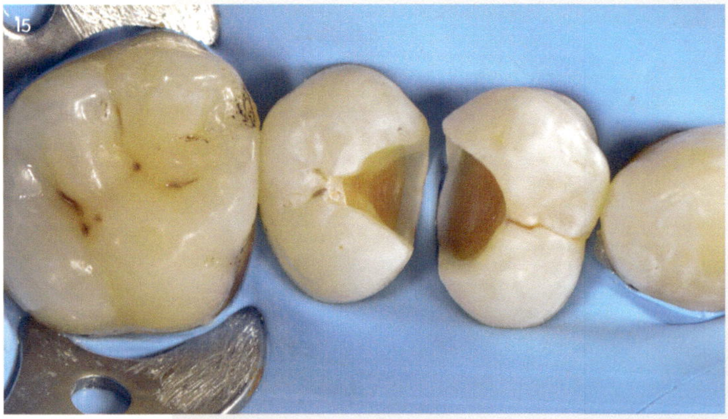

Figure 15 After anesthesia, a rubber dam is applied, and the cavity is prepared with round diamond and round carbide bur with air water coolant.

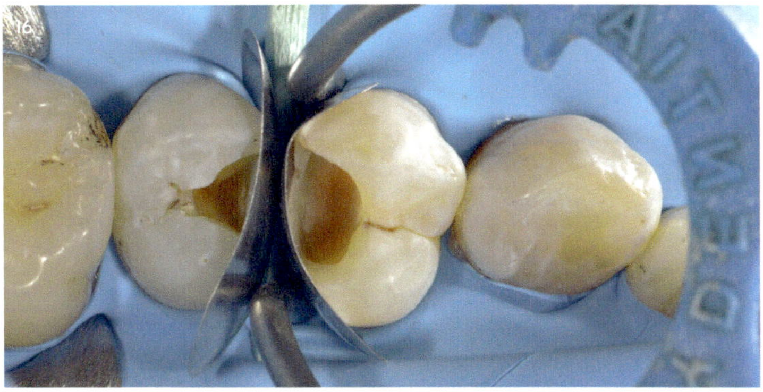

Figure 16 Matrices applied together with a ring to adapt them to the walls, proximal walls are built one at a time, and one matrix is removed after building the wall to ensure a tight contact point.

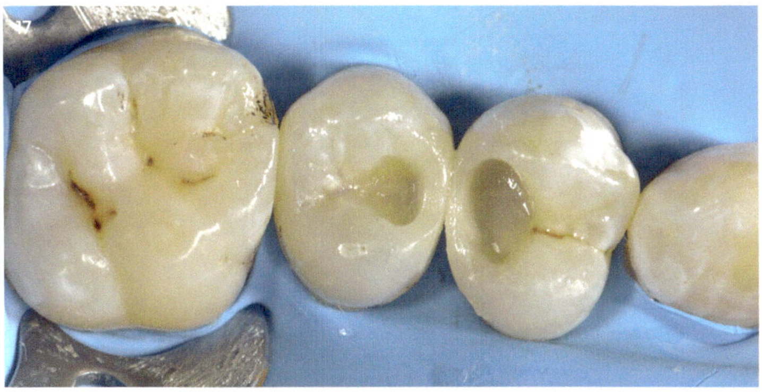

Figure 17 After building up, one by one, all proximal walls, we got easy-to-fill class 1 cavities.

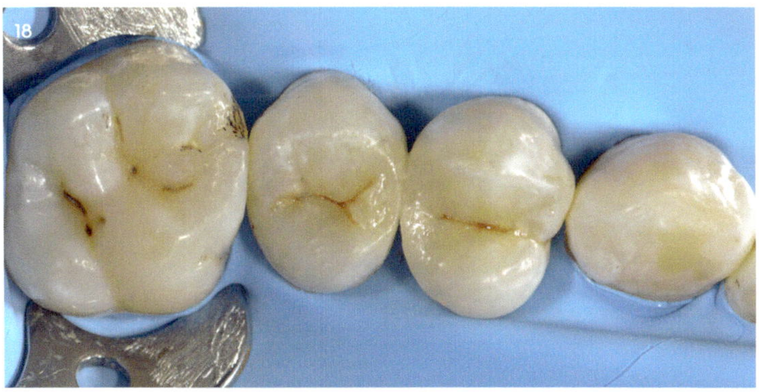

Figure 18 To create final anatomy, body shade composite from Z350(3M) was used.

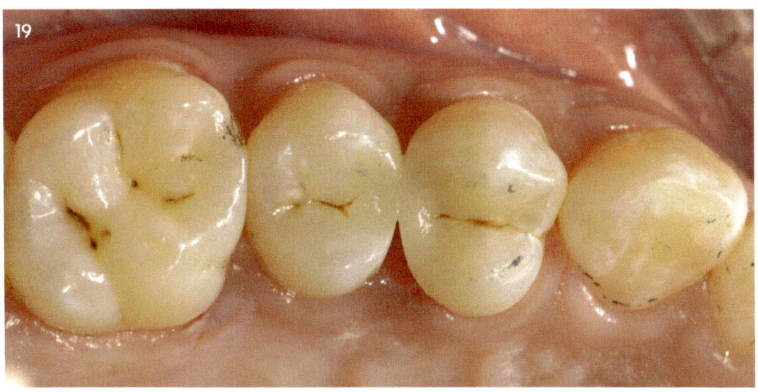

Figure 19 One week follow-up.

Full Quadrant Treatment

Quadrant multiple restorations are very convenient to restore in one single session. When performing multiple restorations, we have access to areas we couldn't reach when proceeding tooth by tooth. Multiple restorations are beneficial to both patients and dental offices for a variety of reasons: the patients benefit from fewer dental appointments and less time away from work, while the office benefits from increased production in fewer visits.

Clinical Case 3 (Pizza Technique)

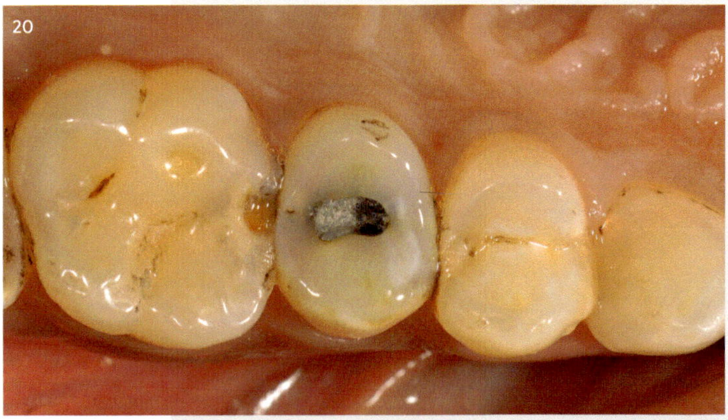

Figure 20 Initial picture of teeth 16, 15, 14 with class 2 decay and poor amalgam filling.

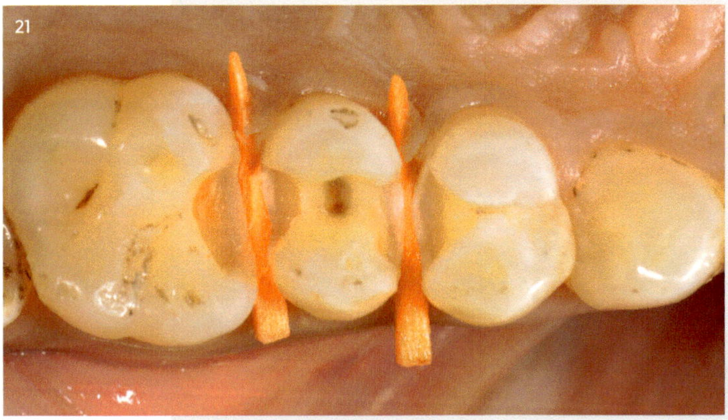

Figure 21 After anesthesia and interproximal wedge placement, cleaning of the caries and refining the enamel with fine grained diamond burs.

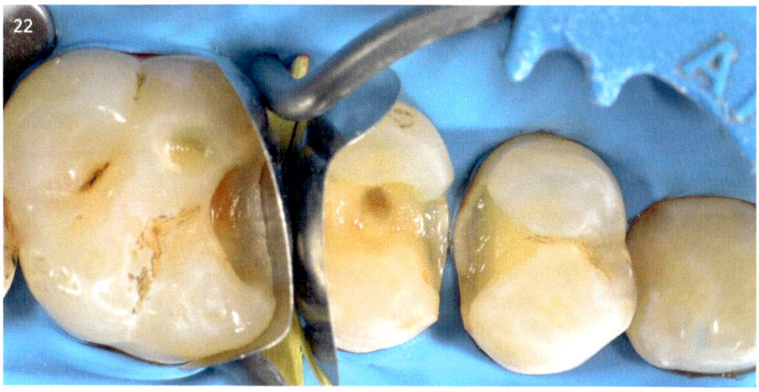

Figure 22 Matrices were placed simultaneously, with the advantage of time saving, and of preventing contamination of cavities during treatment. To allow the matrix to embrace the tooth, we use the rings.

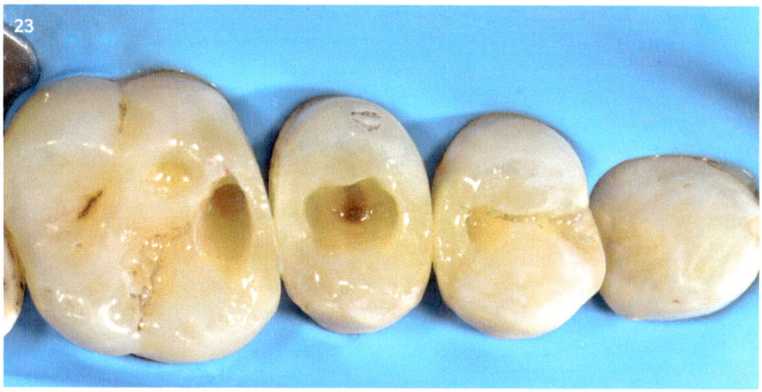

Figure 23 After building up of cavities one by one, we got easy-to-fill class 1 cavities.

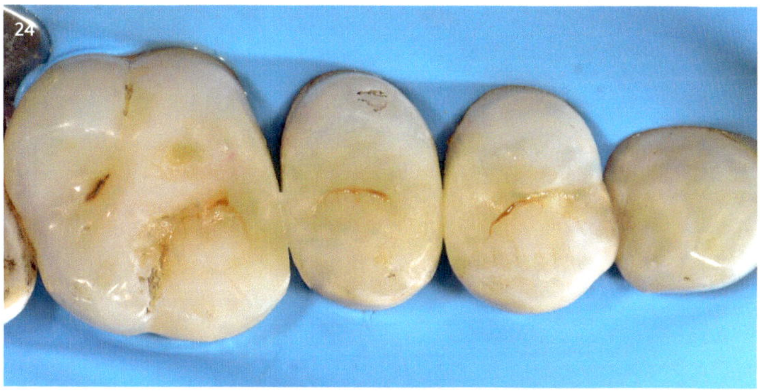

Figure 24 For final anatomy, body shade of Z350 (3M) was used.

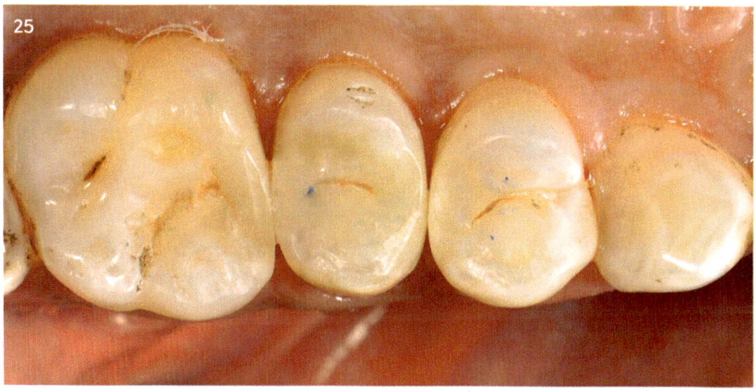

Figure 25 After rubber dam removal, occlusion is adjusted with articulating paper.

Without a doubt, Pizza is an excellent technique that produces good results, and everyone wants to complete their work more quickly without compromising the quality of their work. Recently, some articles about a new technique, the "Espresso Technique", were published in StyleItaliano by Giuseppe Chiodera. I started using this wonderful approach in my exercises and clinical cases and achieved beautiful results quickly.

The Espresso Technique

Designed to be useful in everyday dentistry, the Espresso Technique is basically a tip for shaping the occlusal anatomy altogether, without missing proportions or valuable information which is drawn onto the tooth. In this technique, put the material into the cavity up to 1.5 mm from the cavity edge, in the way you prefer: horizontal, oblique, respecting the C factor. Posterior misura LM Arte can lay on the edge of preparation because of its shape and 1.5 mm thickness that will represent that of the final layer. It is important to be careful to remove all the composite excess and to properly distribute the composite on the margins. Fill the remaining part of cavity with bulk fill or packable composite and compact it with Condensa LM Arte on the entire occlusal surface and lay the Condensa LM Arte instrument on the cusp to copy its inclination. In the same way we also remove the excess material. With the Fissura instrument we can draw the sulci and improve the marginal adaptation of the material to reduce the finishing time and the restoration.

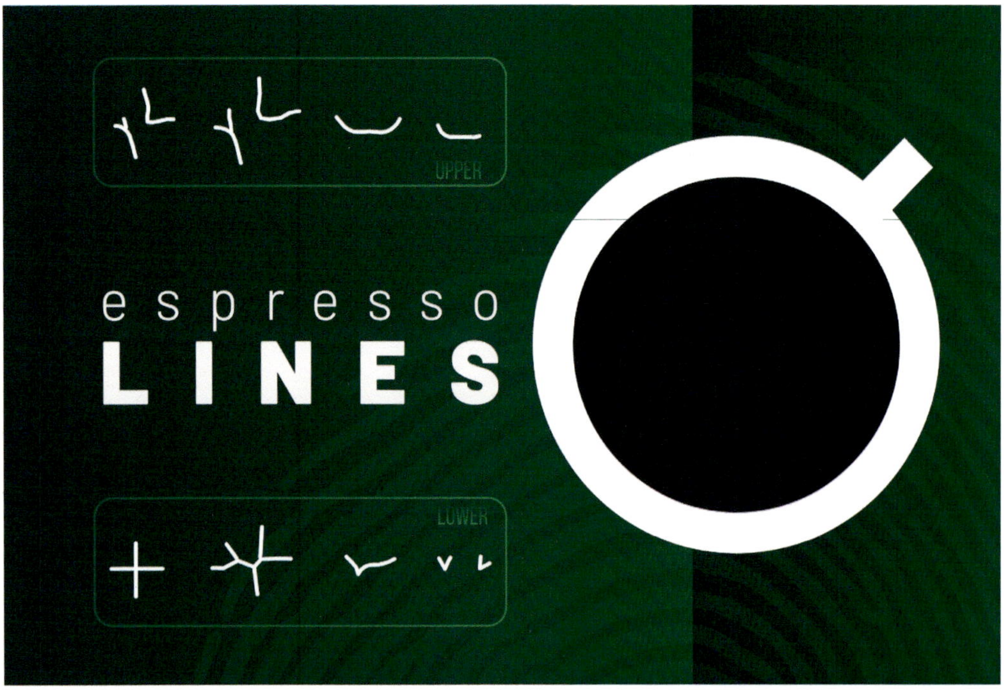

Figure 26 The Espresso technique (StyleItaliano).

Advantages of Espresso Technique

1. It is a fast learning curve.
2. It gives predictable results, without depending on the clinical team's personal skills or the artistic inspiration of the day.
3. It allows you to schedule your agenda more efficiently, as it's faster than traditional layering techniques and doesn't really take much time if more anatomy is lost.

Exercise 5

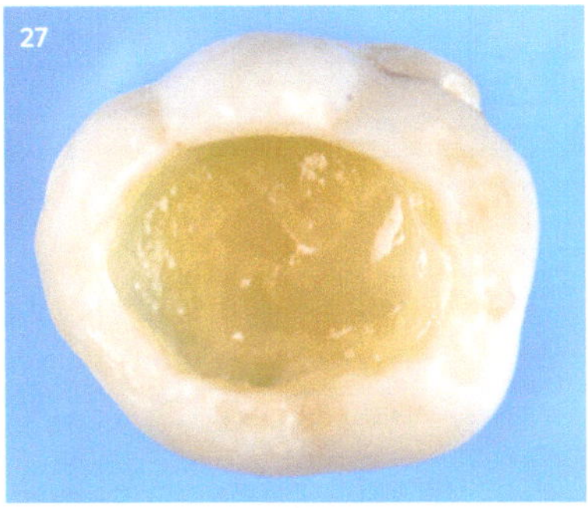

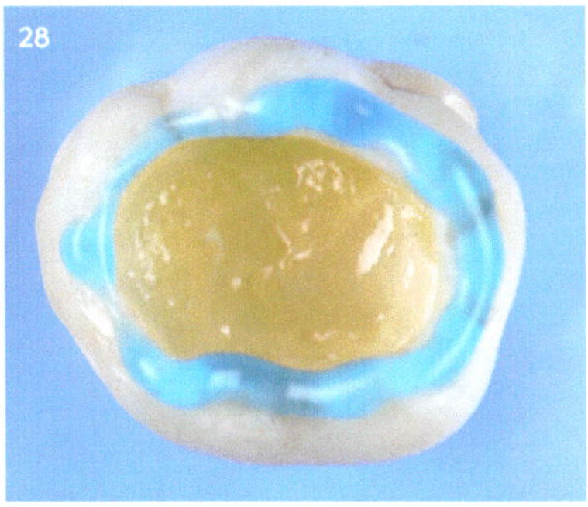

Figure 27 Initial picture of cavity.

Figure 28 Selective etching of the enamel with orthophosphoric acid was performed for 30 seconds.

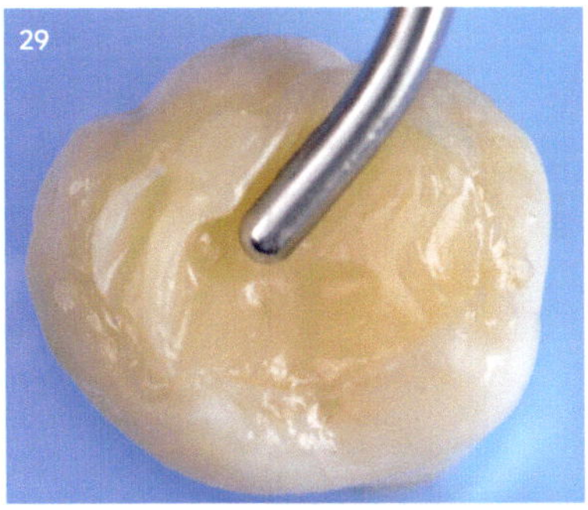

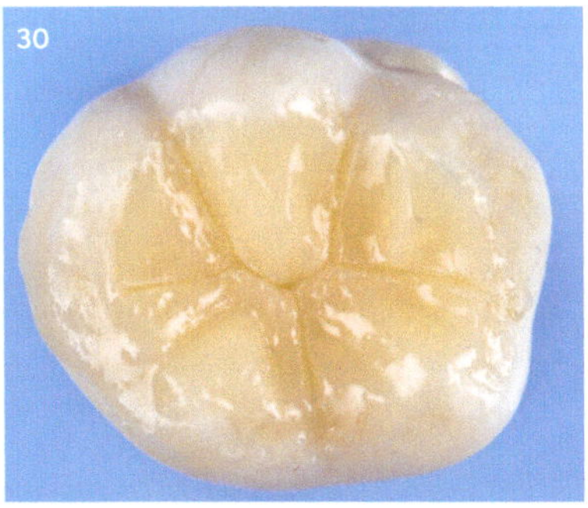

Figure 29 After application and curing of universal adhesive, our next step is to place bulk fill composite. Now we must design our surfaces. First, remove the excess with LM Arte Condensa following cuspal inclination to get shape of the tooth.

Figure 30 As you can see, after having drawn your essential lines, finishing the anatomy is piece of cake.

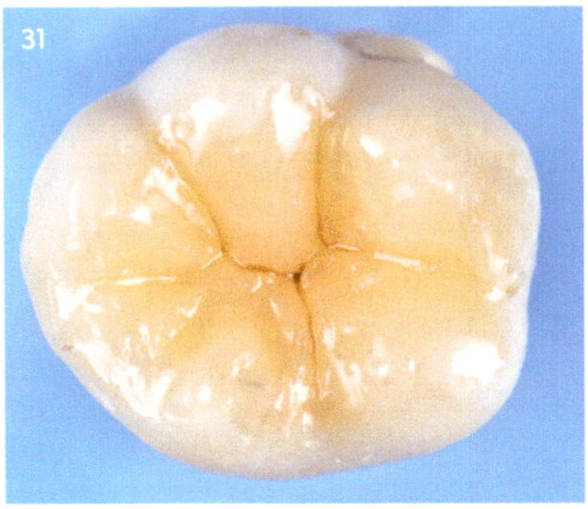

Figure 31 Final image after finishing and polishing with Lucida.

One of the main challenges in daily clinical practice is the replacement of old defective restorations, either due to caries, fracture, or poor esthetics. To do it in a simple and efficient way, we need to know the tooth anatomy, meaning not only the macro and micro morphology but also its internal structure, to imitate it perfectly with different opacities and thickness of composite resins. Modern research is focused on biomaterials, tissue regeneration, stem cells, and healing. Some of these concepts are still science fiction, but we hope just for a short time. At present some great technological advances and research have provided incredible, functional materials that have helped solve some problems, although never as accurately as the natural materials. Each tooth layer has an infinite value; an intact tooth is always our first option before applying any dental material, despite its alleged advantage.

Clinical Case 4 (Espresso Technique)

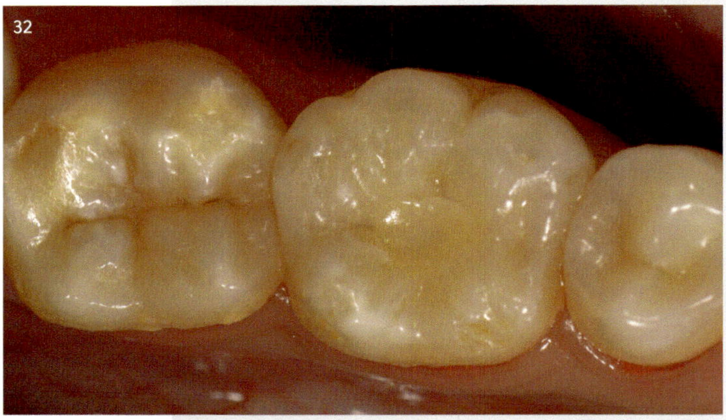

Figure 32 Initial image of tooth with broken down composite restoration. The patient complained of severe sensitivity.

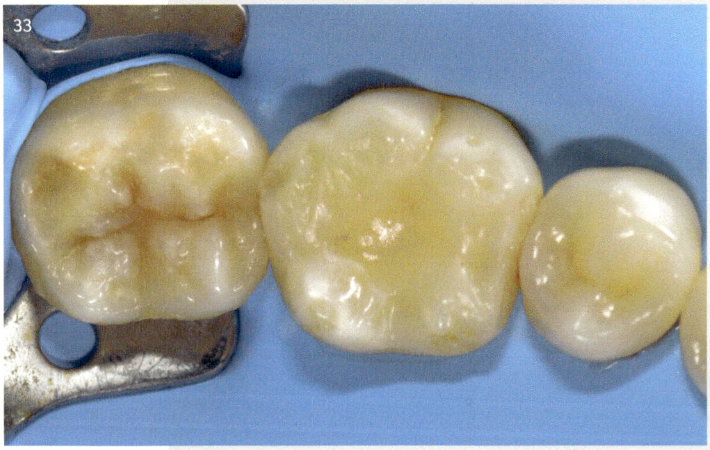

Figure 33 First the operative field was isolated with the rubber dam.

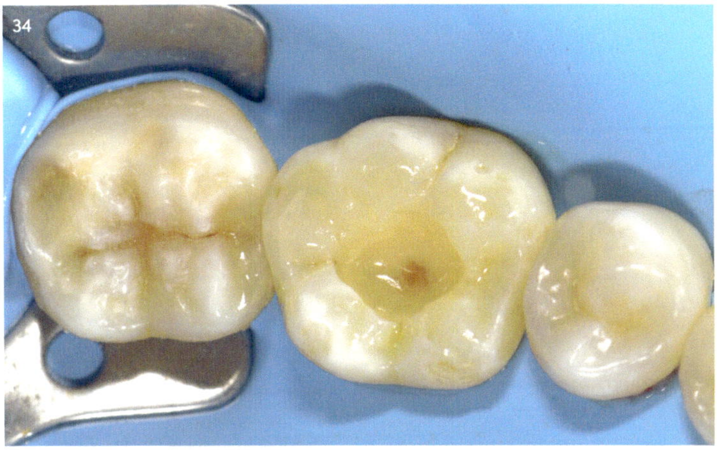

Figure 34 The old restoration was removed and the cavity was properly cleaned.

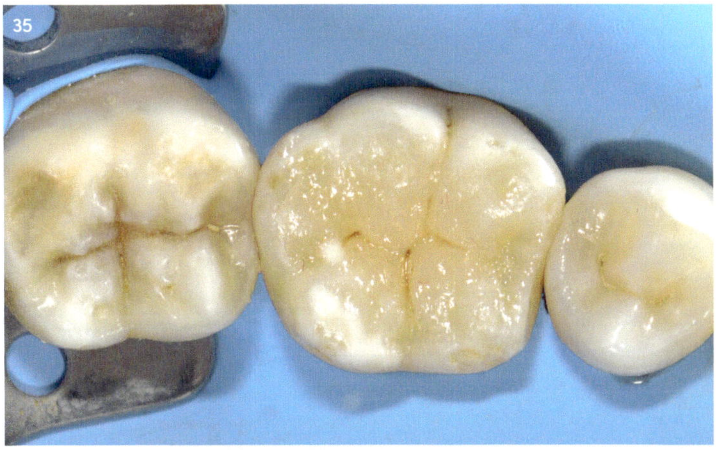

Figure 35 After selective etching of the enamel with orthophosphoric acid and after application of universal adhesive modeling is completed with Espresso Technique.

Figure 36 Image after hydration.

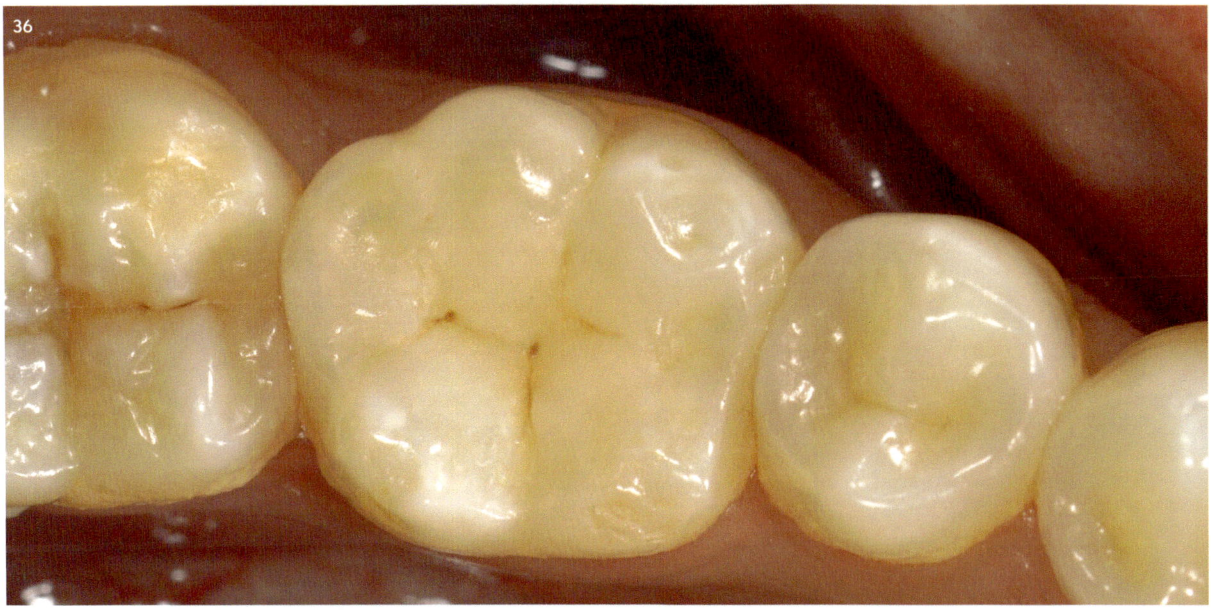

Anatomic Study of Teeth

Understanding of the histology, physiology, and occlusal interactions of the dentitions and supporting tissues is essential for the restorative dentist. Knowledge of the structures of teeth (enamel, dentin, cementum) and their relationship to each other and to the supporting structures is necessary, especially when treating dental caries.
My journey through tooth layers and their analysis will at least give me the knowledge to treat their diseases and mimic their beauty.

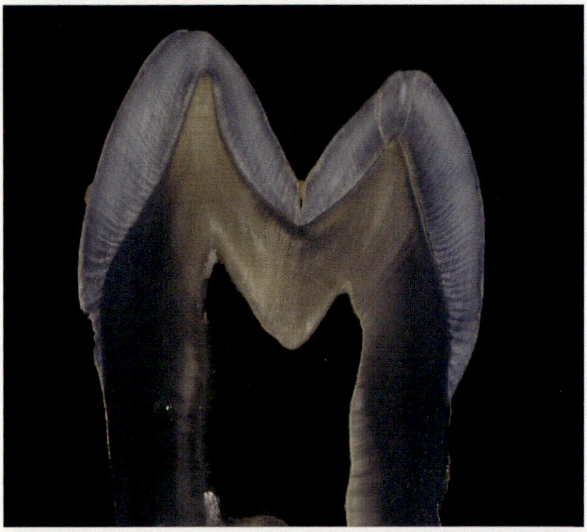

Figure 37 A slice of premolar.

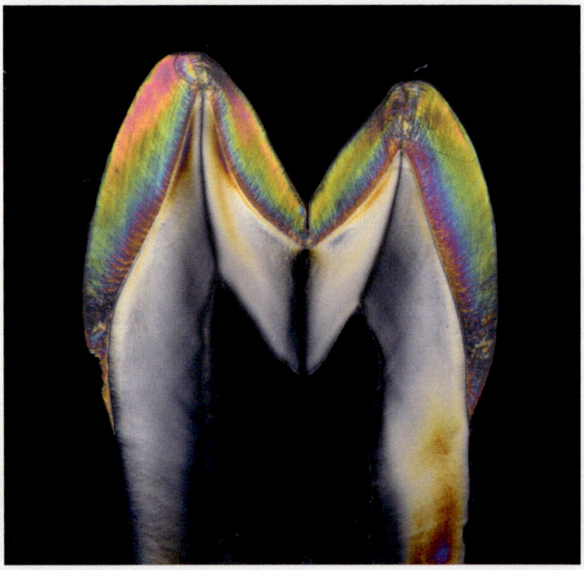

Figure 38 Human enamel and dentin have the property of birefringence, a double reflection.

StyleItaliano Protocols Applied

For perfection in esthetic restoration, we need a precise modeling, right color selection, and good shapes. In order to model the composite precisely, it is suggested to have the right instruments. In the market we can find plenty of suitable instruments for composite stratification. A thin spatula is convenient for precisely modeling the composite, but not all the kits have a thin spatula, maybe because it is a delicate instrument, but the disadvantages outweigh the advantages in the opinion of most of the experts in composites. LM Arte, powered by StyleItaliano, is a wonderful kit for composite modeling, where you can find a thin spatula, thinner than many others in the market.

Clinical Case 5

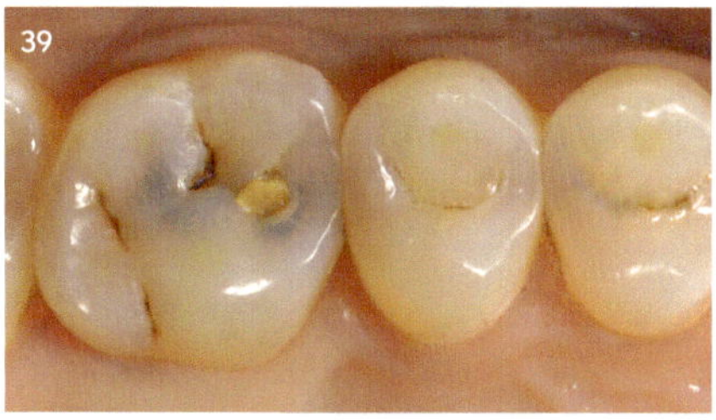

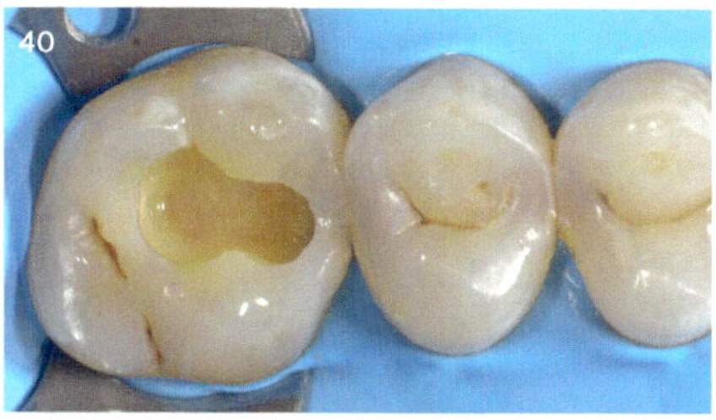

Figure 39 Initial image of tooth.

Figure 40 Cavity preparation and flowable composite at the base of cavity.

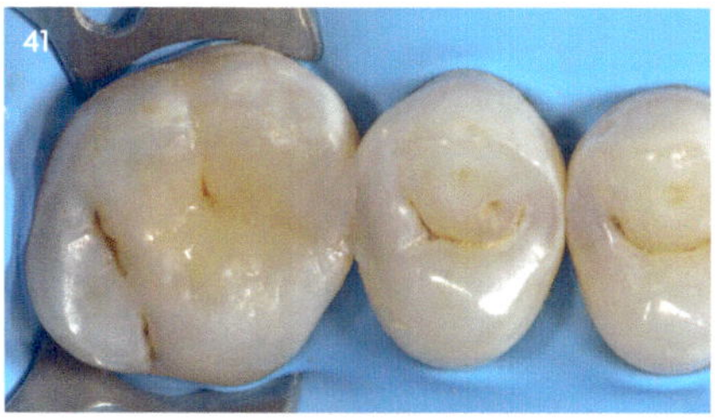

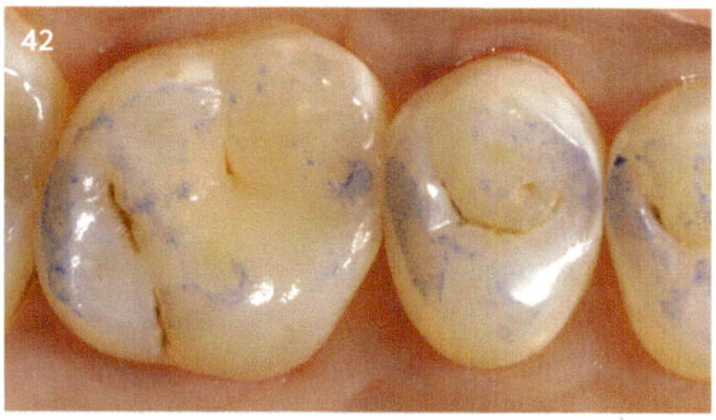

Figure 41 Modeling.

Figure 42 Final image after polishing.

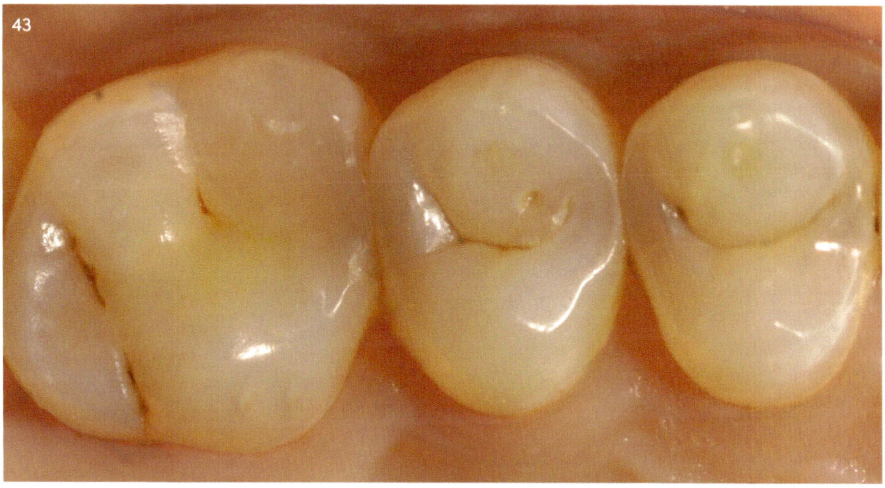

Figure 43 Image after hydration.

The StyleItaliano Group promotes the highest quality dentistry with feasible, repeatable protocols, moderate cost for the patient, while avoiding over-treatments and controlling chair time.

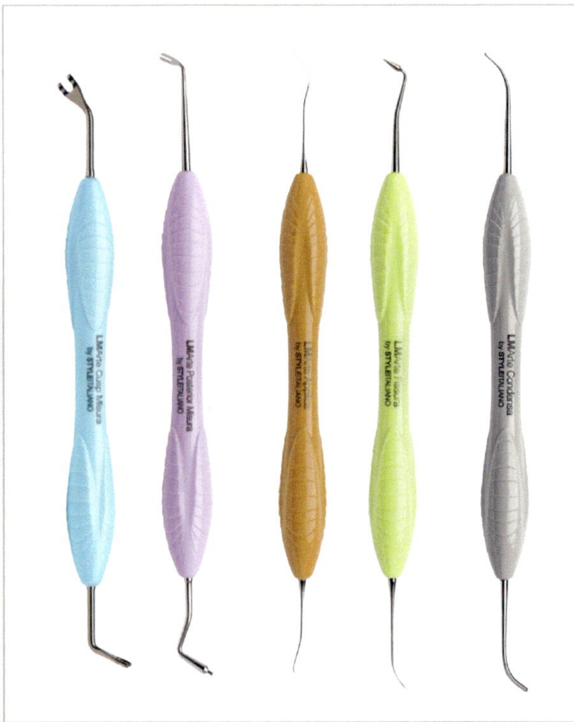

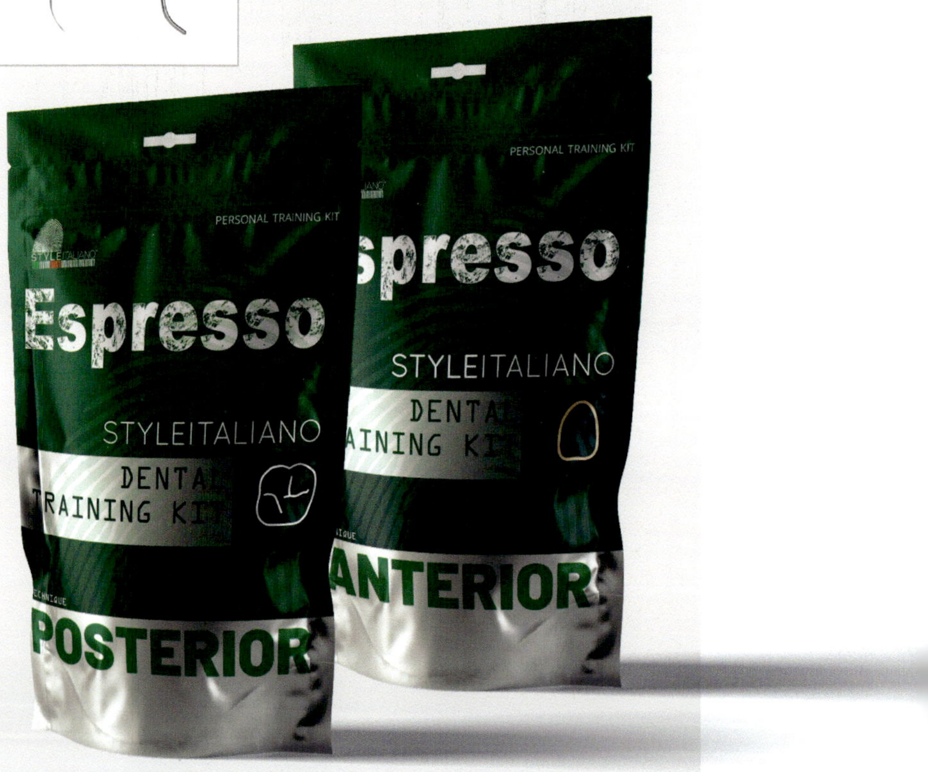

Figure 44 Espresso Mock-Up Anterior and Posterior.

CONCLUSIONS

As time goes by, finding faster and more efficient protocol is becoming more of a necessity. The secret of fabricating esthetic and functional posterior teeth is to generate correct and precise occlusal anatomy. It has been well proven that single shade stratification techniques solve the majority of cases correctly. To achieve a correct anatomy through layering, we propose Pizza and Espresso Technique as well as understanding anatomy, color, thickness, opacity, arrangements, aging, size, shape, orientation, and abnormalities of different layers of teeth and how time plays gracefully with them.

After reading this text we are sure you will learn at least one thing, to love a tooth.

BIBLIOGRAPHY

1. Chiodera G, Orisini G, Tosco v, Manauta J, Devoto W, Putignano A, Essential Line: a simplified filling and modeling technique for direct posterior composite restoration. *Int J Esthet Dent.* 2021;16(2):168-184.
2. Manauta J, Salat A. *Layers. An Atlas of Composite Resin Stratification.* Quintessence pub. 2012.
3. Manauta J, Salat A. *Layers 2, Direct Composites: The StyleItaliano Clinical Secrets.* Quintessence pub. 2022.
4. Hardan L, Sidawi L, Akhundov M, Bourgi R, Ghaleb M, Dabbagh S, Sokolowski K, Suarez C. One-year clinical performance of the Fast-Modeling Bulk Technique and Composite-Up Layering Technique in Class 1 Cavities. *Polymers.* 2021;13:1873.
5. Hein S, Polansky J. *Photography in Dentistry: Unlocking Infinite Creative Possibilities.* Quintessence pub. 2011.
6. Kataoka S, Mjor IA, Nishimura Y. *Nature's Morphology: An Atlas of Tooth Shape and Form.* Quintessence pub. 2002.
7. Magne P, Holz J. Stratification of composite restorations: Systematic and durable replication of natural aesthetics. *Pract Periodontics Aesthet Dent.* 1996;8:61-68.
8. Re D, Cerutti A, Mangani F, Putignano A. *Restauri Estetico-Adesivi Indiretti Parziali nei Settori Posteriori.* UTET. 2007.
9. Sieber C. *Voyage-Visions in Color and Form.* Quintessence pub. 1994.
10. Spreafico R. Direct and semi-direct posterior composite restorations. *Pract Periodontics Aesthet Dent.* 1996;8:703-712.
11. Winter R. Visualizing the natural dentition. *J Esthet Dent.* 1993;5:102-117.
12. Adolfi D. *Natural Esthetics.* Quintessence pub. 2002:83-90.

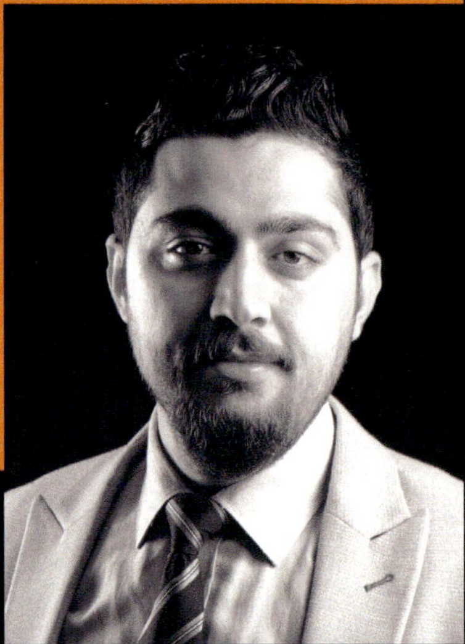

AHMED SAAD

Iraq

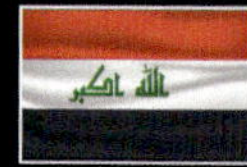

Dr Ahmed Saad received his BDS degree from Tikrit University, College of dentistry in 2014. He earned his Master of Science degree in conservative and aesthetic dentistry from Mustansiriyah University (Iraq) in 2019.

He is working in the field of restorative dentistry at Al-Bayan University, College of dentistry (Iraq) as a lecturer. He is the coordinator of the basic and advanced courses with direct and indirect restorations in dentistry (Baghdad; Iraq).

He is an active member of the Iraqi dental association from 2014.

Dr Saad opened a private dental practice in Baghdad in 2019 and in the same year he achieved his membership from StyleItaliano as a silver member.

Dr Saad is the founder of rivan courses in a private training center established in 2019 that mainly focus on indirect restoration including indirect veneers, crown and bridge and partial restorations courses.

He is a gold and active international StyleItaliano member.

He is the country chairperson for Iraq in the European Society of Cosmetic Dentistry (ESCD).

POSTERIOR INDIRECT OVERLAYS IN STYLEITALIANO PHILOSOPHY

The main purpose of esthetic dentistry is to provide maximum preservation of tooth structure. Further, the development and evolution of adhesive concepts have extensively influenced modern concepts in restorative dentistry including both direct and indirect restorations. The challenge for the partial indirect restoration starts from the case selection and ends with the occlusal compatibility. Ceramic (lithium disilicate glass-ceramic) is the first-choice material in the case of multiple restorations with wide coverage. Long-term intraoral success and the ability to create conservative preparations make bonded porcelain restorations an ideal restorative material in many situations[1-3]. It is important to note that the clinical success of ceramic restorations in posterior teeth after 10 years is 93.5%[4]. On one hand, the advantages[5,6] of adhesively cemented restorations compared to a direct technique consist in creating an ideal anatomy of occlusal surfaces, an excellent control of contact points with healthy emergence profiles, and the possibility of occlusal evaluation by means of an articulator. Partial indirect posterior restoration is highly indicated in class II cavities of large dimensions with unsupported axial walls. The presence of cracks in enamel and dentin (in vital teeth), and the absence of marginal ridges in endodontically treated teeth requires total coverage even in the presence of residual walls with adequate thickness[7,8,9].

DISCUSSION AND CLINICAL CASE

Build-Up

To provide a correct geometry of the cavity and to produce an optimal thickness of the restoration, the build-up must be performed to fill the undercuts created during caries removal. Moreover, to put the margin of the preparation at accessible and repairable area for the laboratory work and for the cementation.

The immediate dentin sealing (IDS) and the filling of the undercut by flowable resin materials play multiple roles, including the reinforcement of cavity walls. It simultaneously eliminates undercuts and saves tooth structure and, if needed, permits the occlusal relocation of cervical margins. Finally, it offers a physical and biological protection during the temporary phase (eliminating virtually all possible biological complications, such as tooth sensitivity and bacterial leakage), leading to a markedly improved protocol comparing to the "traditional" approach for adhesive indirect restorations. At the time of cementation, it will also act as a physical barrier against the mechanical surface treatment (sandblasting) of the cavity, therefore preserving the integrity of the sealed dentin surfaces[10].

In case of deep cervical margins without biological width violation, it is clinically convenient to move the margins coronally, applying a layer of highly reinforced flowable composite (1 to 1.5 mm thick). When the position of cervical margins does not allow for the correct isolation with rubber dam or there is a biological width violation, a surgical approach is necessary.

Preparation Design

Preparation starts with the removal of the existing restoration and decayed tissues without finishing the enamel margins. In less accessible areas (usually interproximally), selectively diamond coated instruments facilitate the preparation and the finishing of the cavity.

Fissures (in dentin or enamel) should ideally be included in the preparation, considering potential bacterial leakage or structural weakening, although their extension in inaccessible zones often prevents these flaws from being fully eliminated.

Generally, if the cusp thickness of the vital tooth is <2 mm, a cusp coverage is suggested, while for the non-vital posterior teeth, the thickness limit is 3 mm. For the cusp thickness evaluation and wall thickness, dental vernier (caliper) instrument (📷 1), and the LM Arte cusp misura (LM-Dental, Finland) instrument could be helpful (📷 2).

For the LM Arte cusp misura (LM-Dental, Finland) instrument: if the forked instrument tip penetrates up to its marks, the tooth structure is too weak to withstand occlusal forces without being deflected, so the reduction must be considered according to the clinical situation (📷 3).

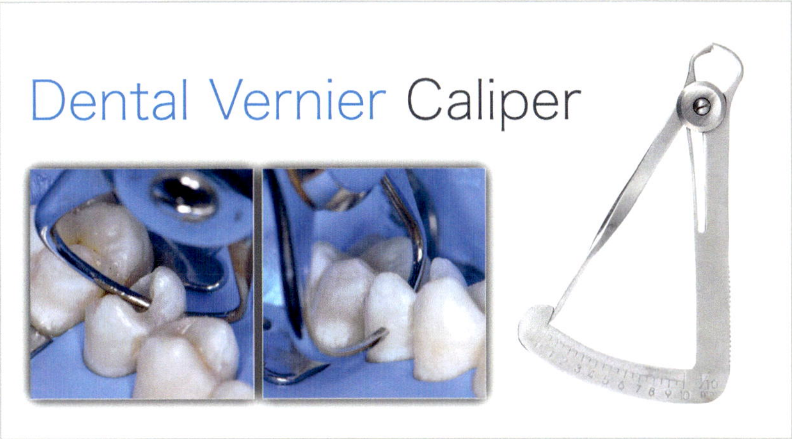

Figure 1 Dental vernier (caliper) instrument used for the cusp thickness evaluation.

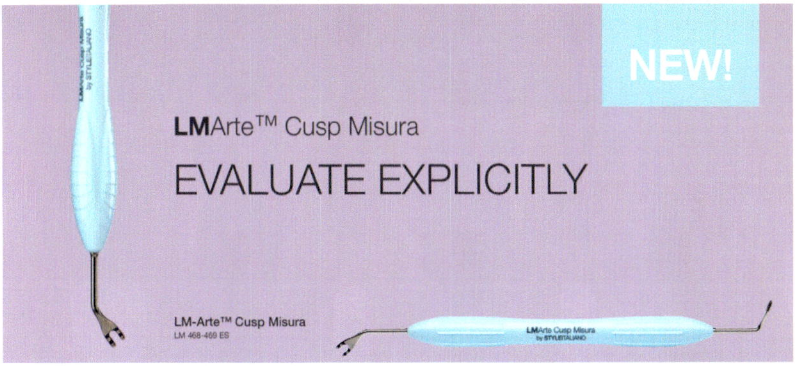

Figure 2 The LM Arte cusp misura (LM-Dental, Finland), instrument used for the cusp thickness estimation.

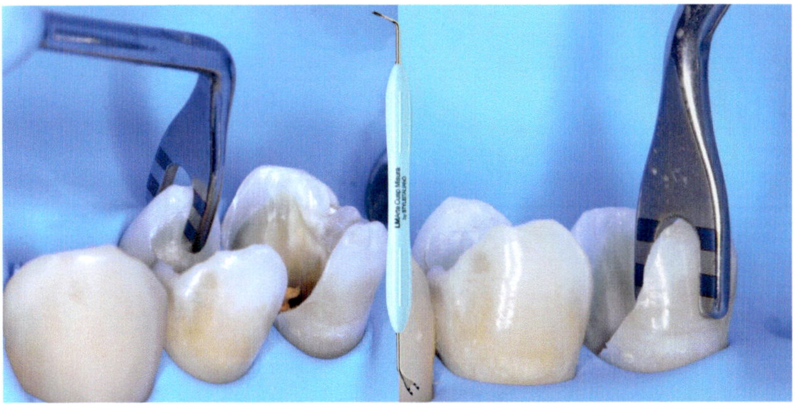

Figure 3 Evaluation and measuring of the cusp thickness and height by means of the LM Arte cusp misura (LM-Dental, Finland).

ALWAYS TRY TO PUT YOUR MARGIN BELOW THE CONTACT POINT WITH THE ADJACENT TEETH MESIALLY AND DISTALLY TO FACILITATE THE INSERTION OF PROSTHESIS AND TO REMOVE THE EXCESS OF CEMENT; IN ADDITION TO THIS, A NEW HEALTHY CONTACT AREA WILL BE CREATED.

It is recommended a minimum of 2 mm as minimal wall width/thickness before reinforcement. In cases where the minimal residual thickness is below this measurement, a cusp coverage is indicated. The aim is to have a more homogeneous biting force distribution, and to offer a "protective effect" for the underlying weakened tooth structure. Occlusal coverage is recommended for cavity walls of 1 mm or thinner, while for "intermediate" thickness (1 to 2 mm), the occlusal context including tooth position, presence of parafunctions, and the kind of lateral guidance (canine or group guidance) should be taken into account when making the therapeutic decision. The cavity configuration, in particular the presence or absence of the marginal ridges, can also play a role in the final strength of the residual walls, especially in endodontically treated teeth[11].
After caries and/or failed restoration removal, a cavity with slightly occlusal divergent walls (5° to 15°), and round internal angles is prepared by using cylindrical round-ended diamond burs.
IDS is a strategy in which a dentin bonding agent is applied to freshly cut dentin and polymerized before making an impression.

Supragingival margins facilitate the impression making, the definitive restoration placement, and the detection of secondary caries. The resulting "invasiveness" could, however, increase the risk of irreversible tooth fracture (below the cemento-enamel junction—CEJ), as is shown in vitro by Fennis et al[12], although such clinical observation is extremely rare in

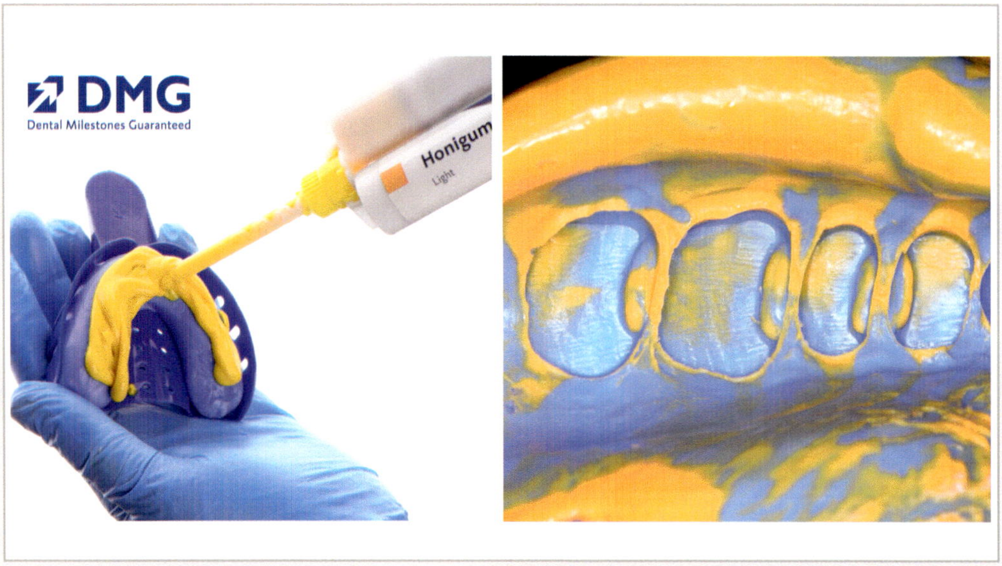

Figure 4 Retraction paste and final impression with laboratory work.

vital teeth. Finally, the systematic occlusal coverage of functional and/or non-functional cusps is not yet advocated, as it is seemingly not proven to increase the final strength of the tooth restoration system, both for composite resins and ceramics[13-14].

Final Impression

When the cavity is ready for impression taking, undercuts must be eliminated or filled with composite (restorative or flowable) during the composite lining. The margins of the cavity especially cervical ones, must be relocated occlusally (at least 0.5 mm over the free gingival margin) to facilitate impression and rubber dam application. Do not over-elevate the margins in order to obtain an optimal, natural proximal emergence profile of the future restoration.

Absence of contact between the cavity and the adjacent teeth should guarantee a good flow of the impression material in the interproximal areas, and make optical impression recording easier. The suitable interocclusal space for the selected restoration material is checked after rubber dam removal in centric and in lateral movements.

The use of an elastomer material such as polyvinylsiloxane (VPS) or polyether is recommended, although polyether materials are rather sensitive to the possible persistence of an oxygen-inhibited layer, which may affect their setting reaction[15] (📷 4). Further, digital (intra-oral scanner) technique can be used for the final impression (📷 5).

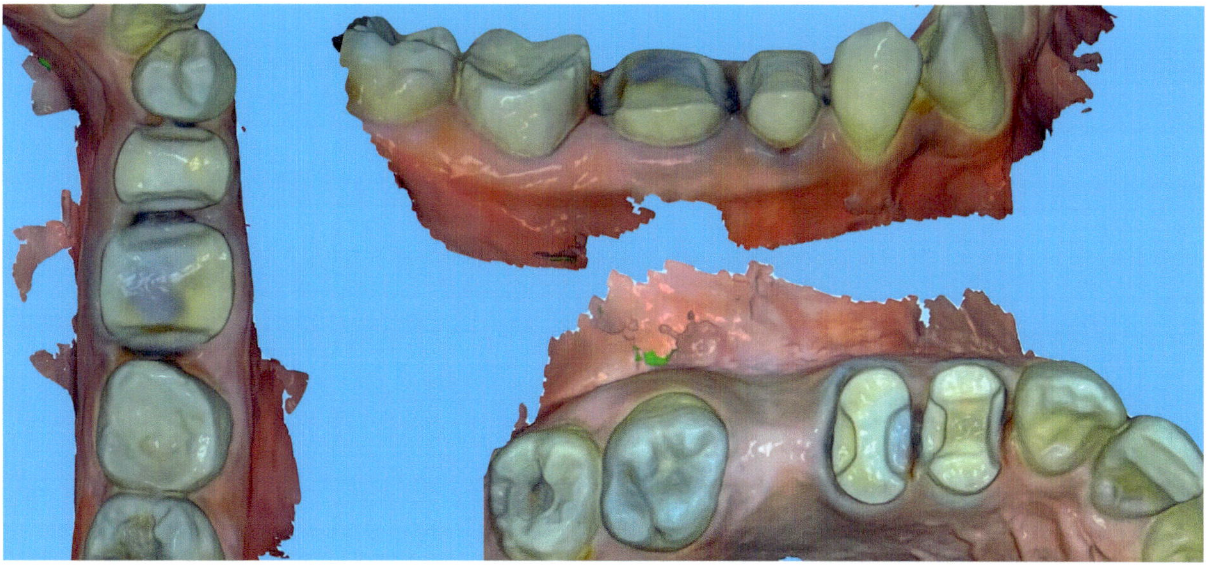

Figure 5 Digital impressions for overlays preparation by using intra-oral scanner.

Cementation

For this kind of non-retentive indirect restoration, the technique for cementation and the material that is being used are critical and must be perfectly executed; any deficiency in this step can compromise the durability of the restoration, and a special surface treatment of the overlay in steps (6) should be done as follows:

- **A.** Hydrofluoric acid 9% for 20 seconds for micro-undercuts and increasing the surface area of lithium disilicate
- **B.** Phosphoric acid 37% for 60 seconds (optional step) to remove the salts and debris (for extra cleaning if contaminated)
- **C.** Silane (Bifunctional molecule that promotes adhesion via covalent bonds with hydroxyl groups)
- **D.** Bonding agent for chemical and micro mechanical retention
- **E.** Cement (Light, Chemical or Dual Cure), with the help of veneer ME (Smile Line, Switzerland) from smile line that powered by StyleItaliano to facilitate the daily work (7)

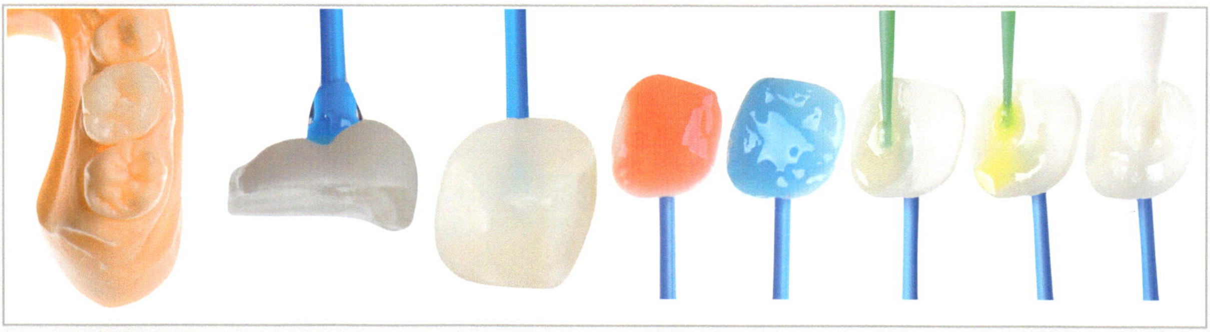

Figure 6 Steps of surface treatment.

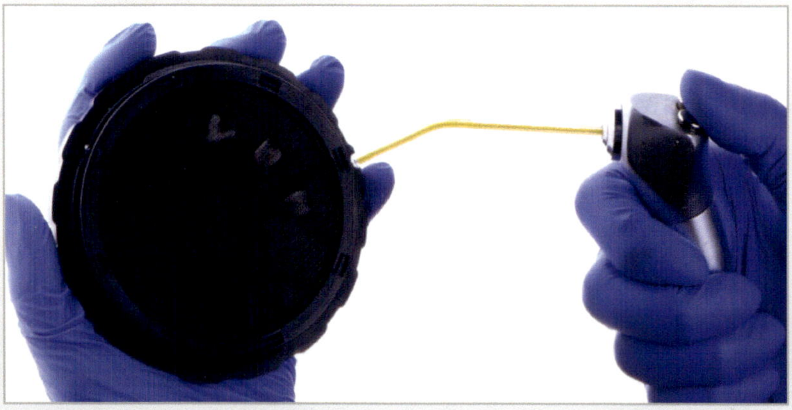

Figure 7 Veneer ME (Smile Line, Switzerland) for overlays surface treatment.

The polymerization shrinkage for cement remains one of the major problems in indirect restorative dentistry. Polymerization shrinkage is affected by several factors, such as resin cement characteristics, cavity configuration factor (C-factor), preparation geometry, cement thickness, and adhesive substrate. Therefore, cement volume is important, in fact, it can increase shrinkage stress regardless the decreased C-factor. Although there is no consensus on the optimal cement spacing, a spacing between 50–100 μm has shown good performance.

The curing methods are a factor in dictating the potential uses of the cements. For example, in cases where very little or no light-cure is possible, chemical-cure cement is the better choice than either a dual-cure or, of course, a light-cure cement.

At the starting of the cementation process, the temporization material is being removed and the tooth is cleaned by pumice and brushes, then chlorohexidine is applied to disinfect the surface. The tooth surface (enamel and composite build-up) treatment should follow these steps (📷 8):

A. Isolation and protection of adjacent teeth proximally by Teflon

B. Sandblasting with aluminum oxide powders

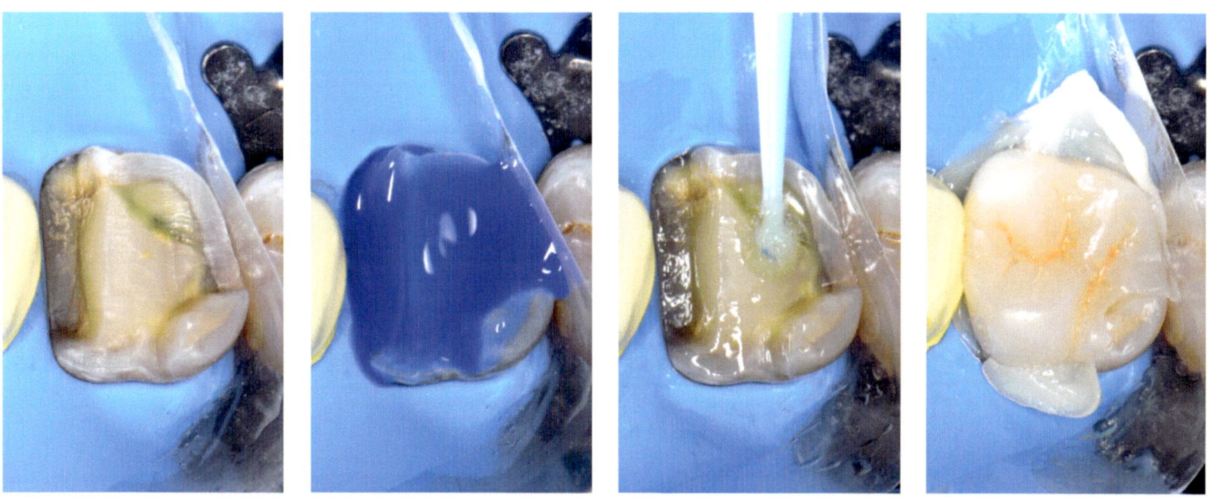

Figure 8 Steps of tooth treatment and ceramic cementation.

C. Total etching 37% phosphoric acid for 20-30 seconds
D. Rinsing
E. Bonding agent on all the area
F. Cementing the prosthesis on the tooth
G. Removing the excess cement
H. Light curing for 20-40 seconds from different direction

Roughening the composite area of adhesion by sandblasting could be helpful to clean and reactivate the composite before the cementation (9) and (10).

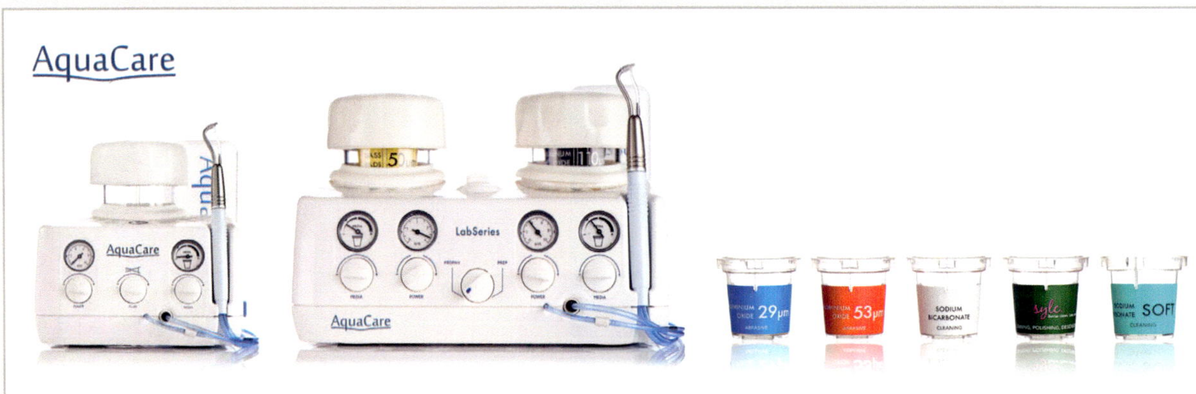

Figure 9 Aquacare Velopex and powders.

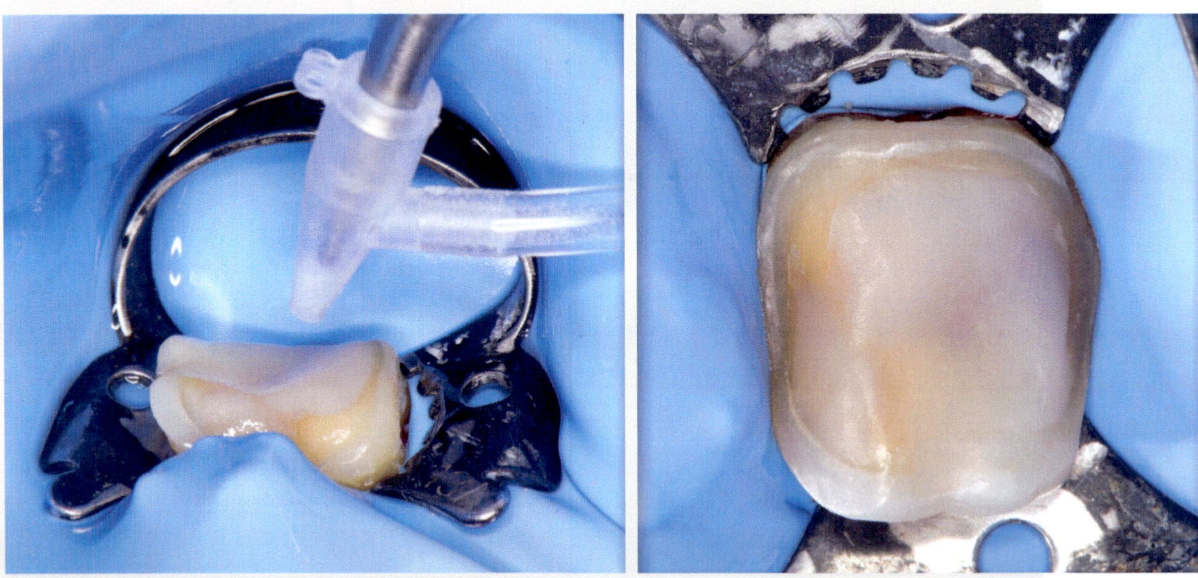

Figure 10 Sandblasting before cementation.

Clinical Case 1

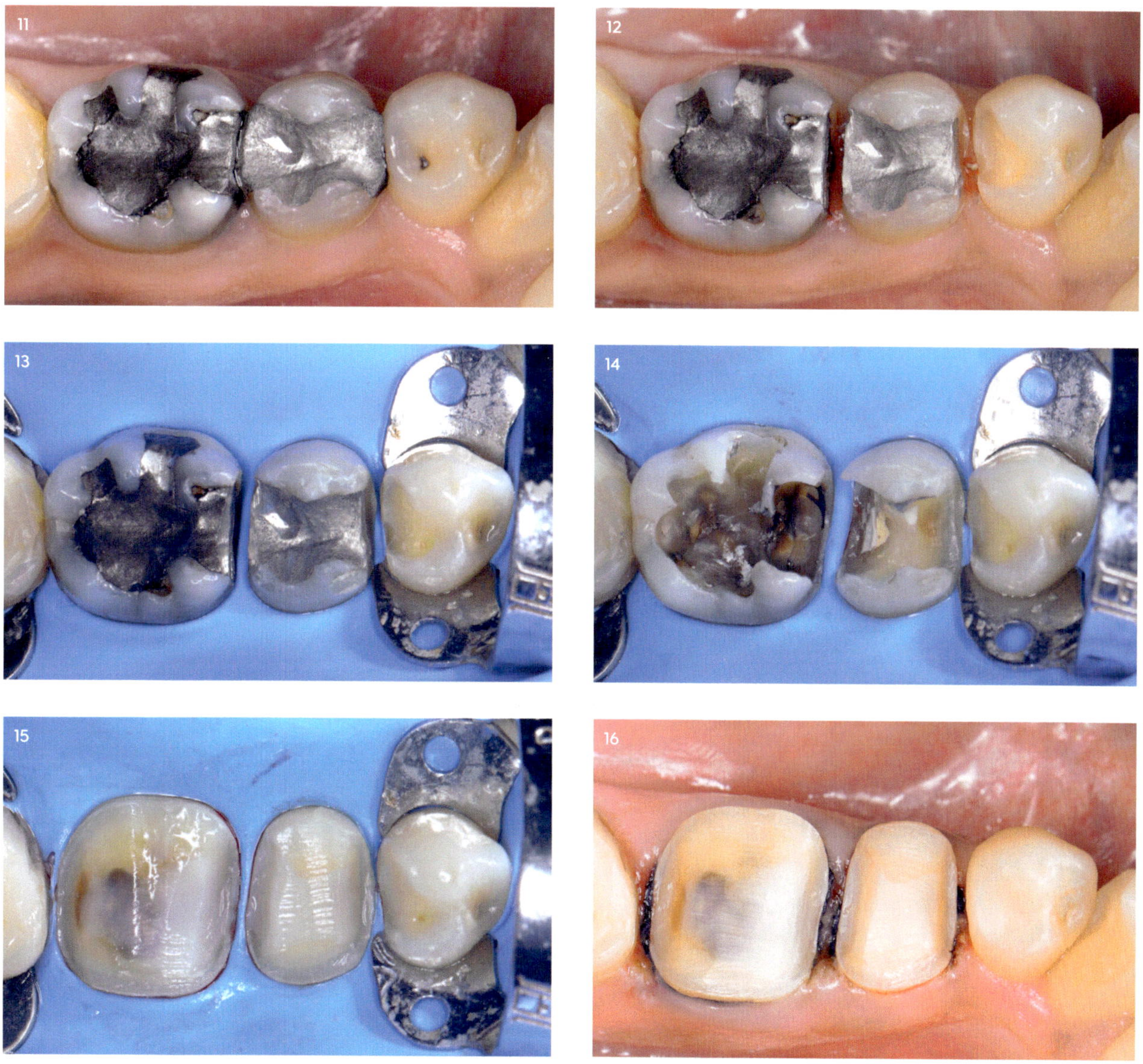

Figure 11 Wide inadequate amalgam restorations with residual and recurrent caries. The teeth was asymptomatic.

Figure 12 Opening the contact area to facilitate the placement of rubber dam.

Figure 13 After rubber dam application.

Figure 14 Amalgam was removed.

Figure 15 Thorough caries cleansing with vitality maintenance of the tooth without pulp exposure, cavity design definition (after adhesive build-up) for overlay with inclined planes of the axial walls, and connection on ramp with box.

Figure 16 Cavities have detailed sharp margins, no undercuts, accessibility of subgingival margins, and no contact with adjacent teeth.

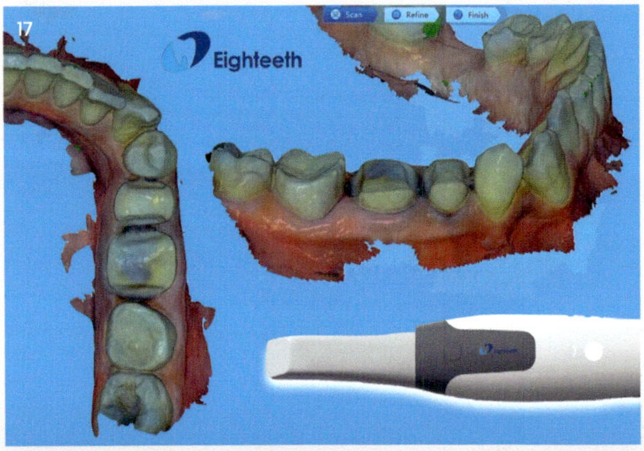

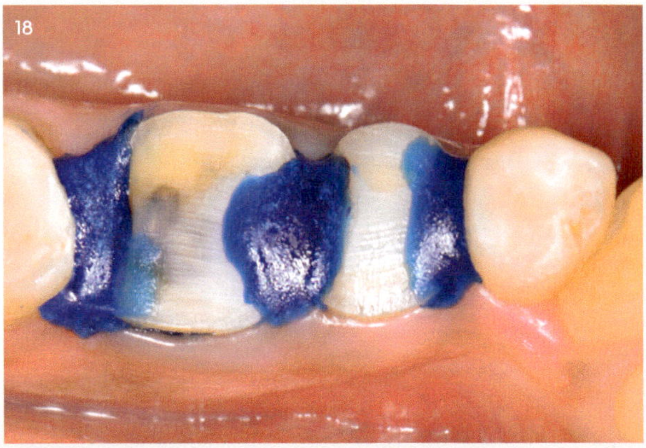

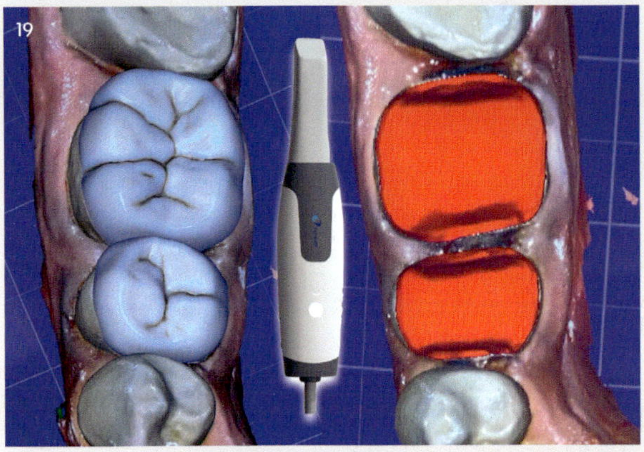

Figure 17 The digital intra-oral scanner (Helios 600 by Eighteeth, Changzhou, China) used for recording. The complete scan was then sent to the laboratory.

Figure 18 Liquid dam used as a provisional.

Figure 19 A digital scan was taken. Here you can see a screenshot from the standard tessellation language (STL) file and details of the preparation without the high definition.

Figure 20 A pressed lithium disilicate overlay was fabricated, then colored and polished.

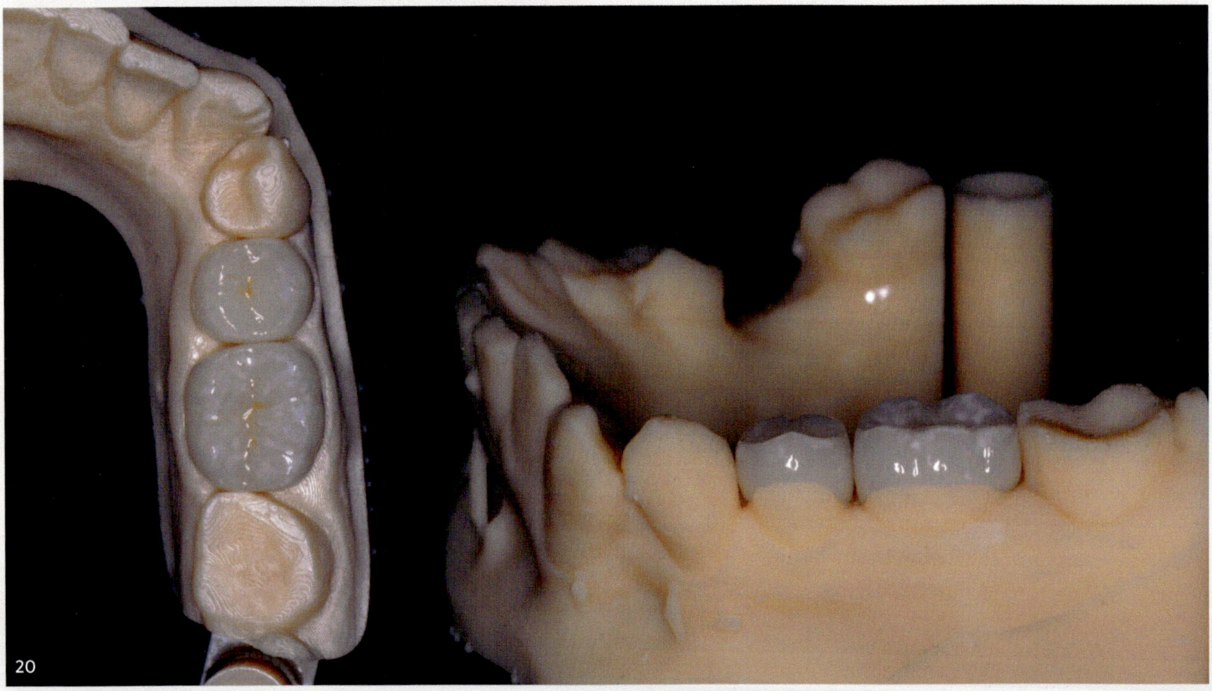

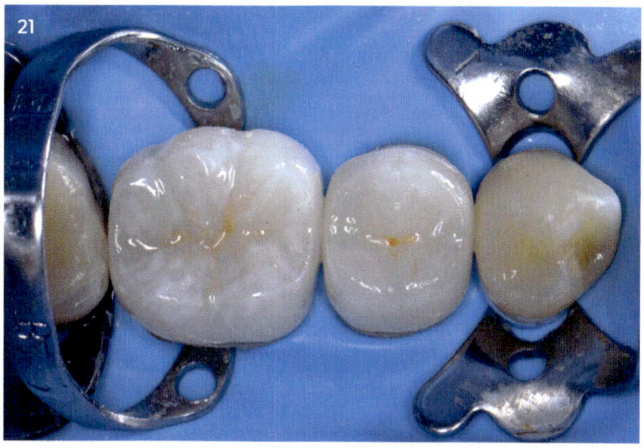

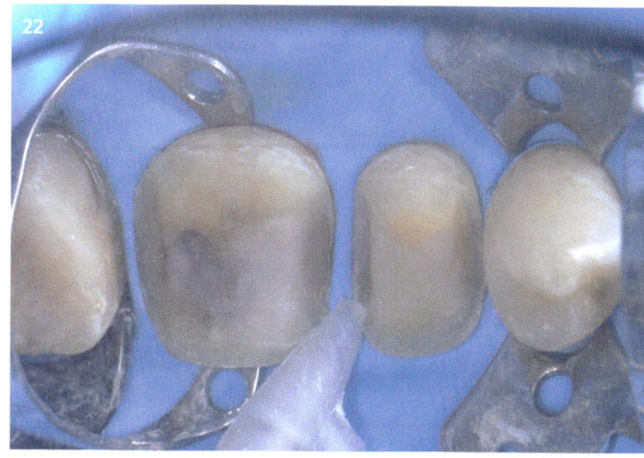

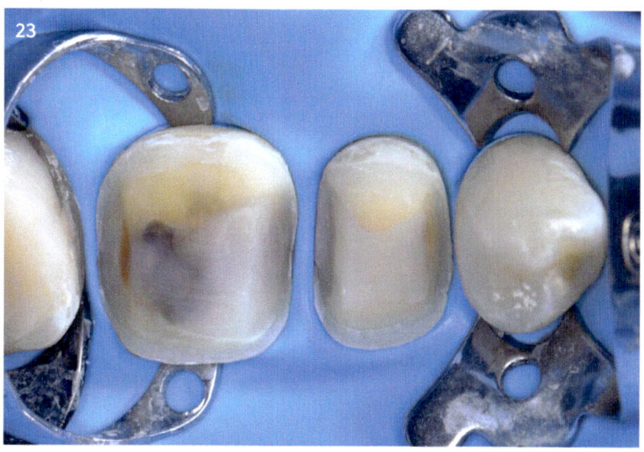

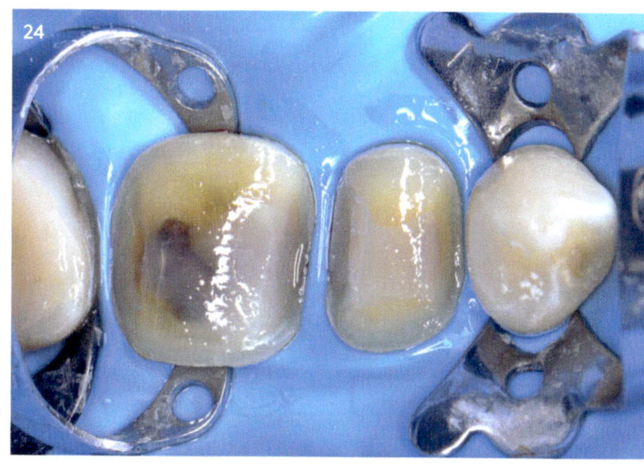

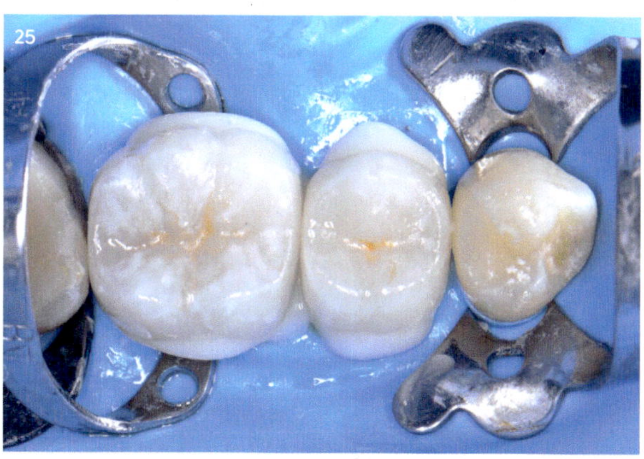

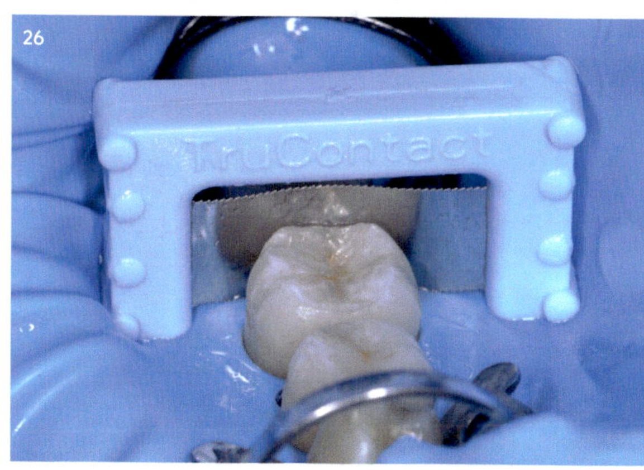

Figure 21 The try-in stage is very important to check the adaptation of the prosthesis before the surface treatment of the lithium disilicate.

Figure 22 Sandblasting of the entire surface using aluminum oxide (53-micron particles) to clean and reactivate the tooth structure and composite.

Figure 23 After sandblasting, teeth were perfectly clean and ready for the bonding procedures.

Figure 24 Application of the bonding agent: in this case the ScotchBond™ Universal (3MEPE, USA) was applied which can be used as a self-etch or as a total-etch technique. The bonding agent is rubbed for 20 seconds.

Figure 25 After injecting resin cement inside the restoration.

Figure 26 The TruContact by Bioclear to remove the excess cement from the contact.

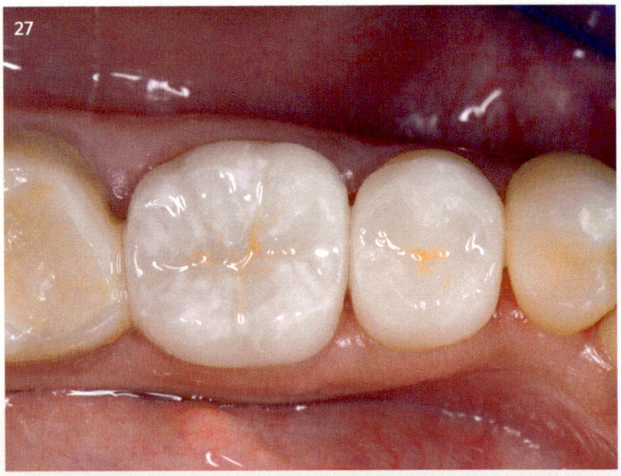

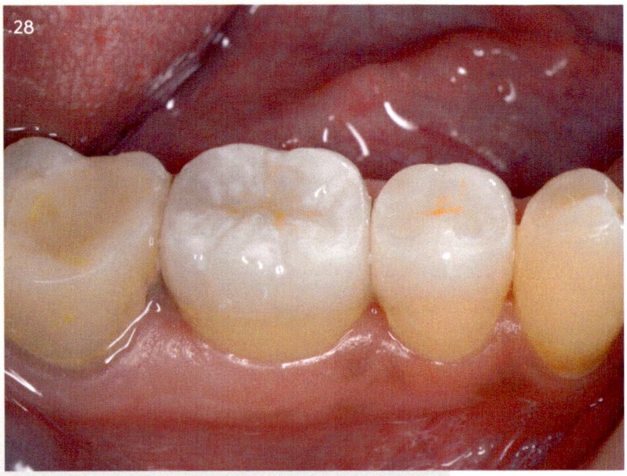

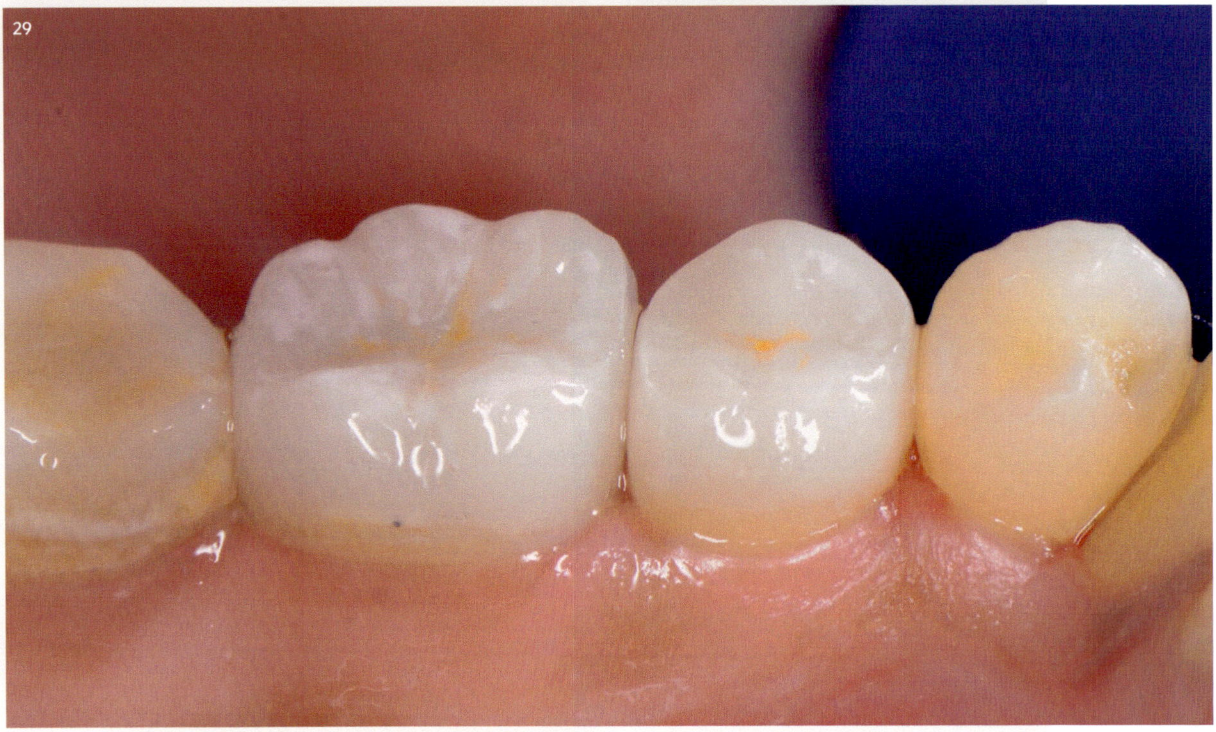

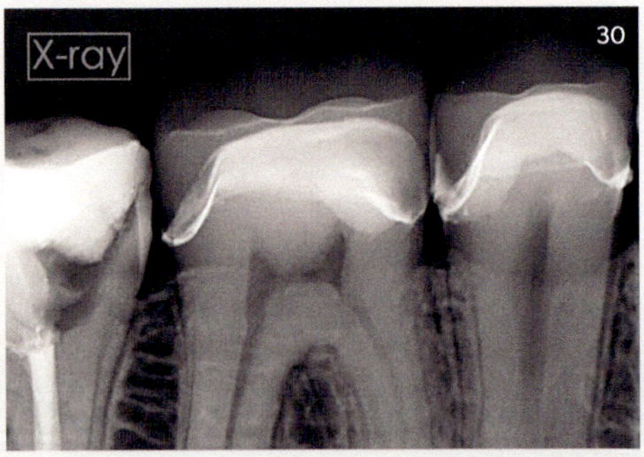

Figure 27 The finished case at the end of the procedure.

Figure 28 At check-up, 10 days later.

Figure 29 Final view of the integrated restorations.

Figure 30 Periapical X-ray.

Clinical Case 2

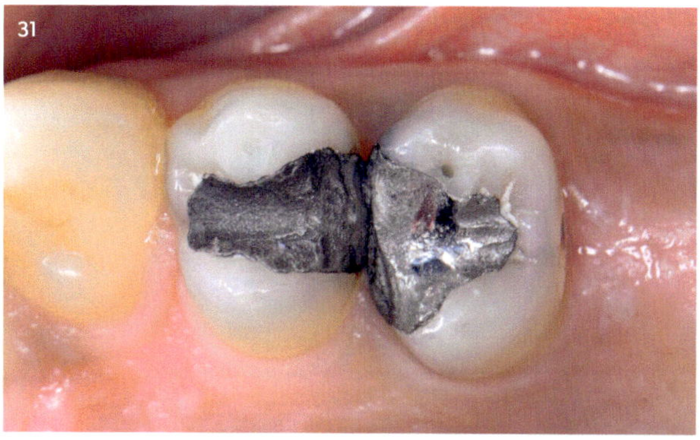

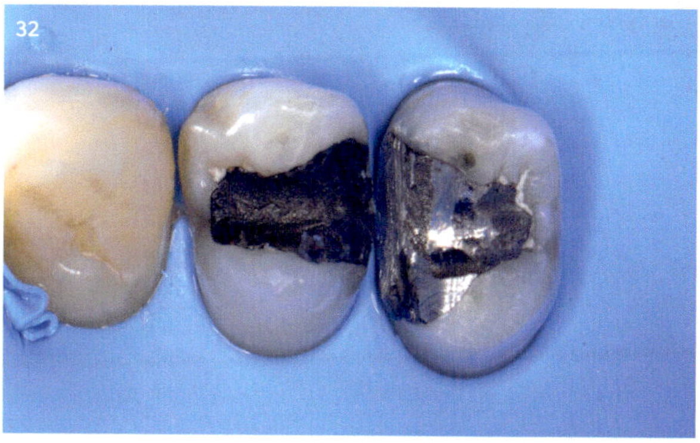

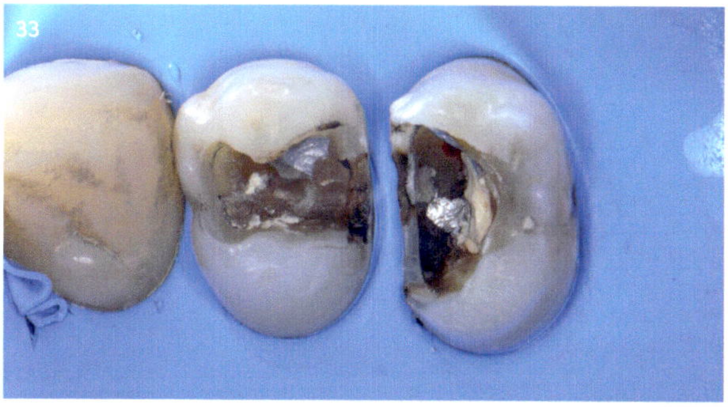

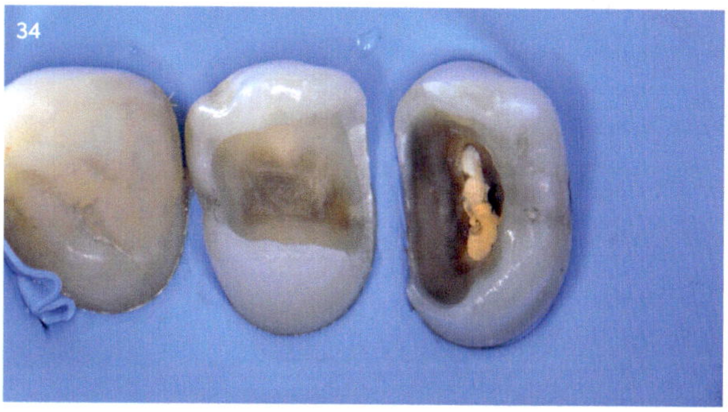

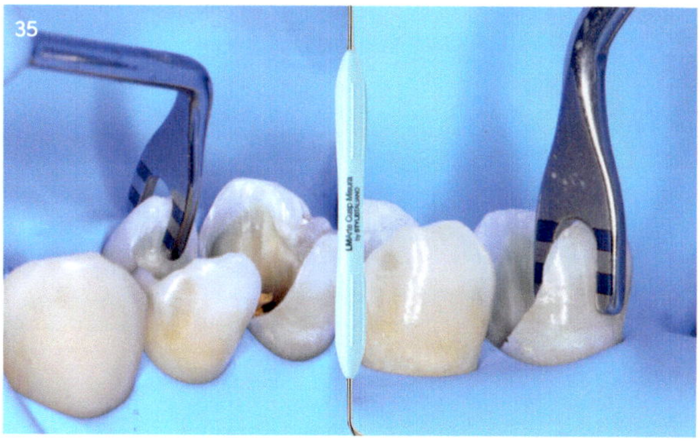

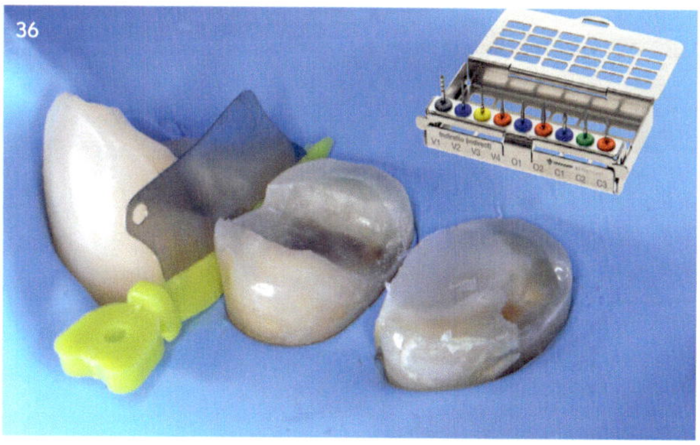

Figure 31 Initial situation of both premolars with amalgam restorations.

Figure 32 Isolation with rubber dam (Nic Tone Dental Dam, thick, mint, MDC dental, Zapopan, Mexico) was done before amalgam removal according to ADA's protocols.

Figure 33 The amalgam was removed first.

Figure 34 Maxillary bicuspid, thin walls of first one and the other one is endodontically treated with a deep mesio-occlusal (MO) cavity. There is a need for a complete cuspal coverage to preserve it from fracture.

Figure 35 Before proceeding, the cusp was measured by means of the LM Arte cusp misura (LM-Dental, Parainen, Finland) to choose the final cavity configuration.

Figure 36 Place the FenderWedge to protect the adjacent tooth.

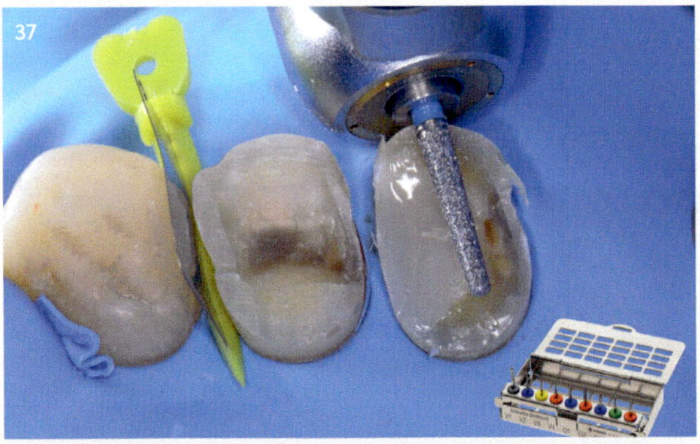

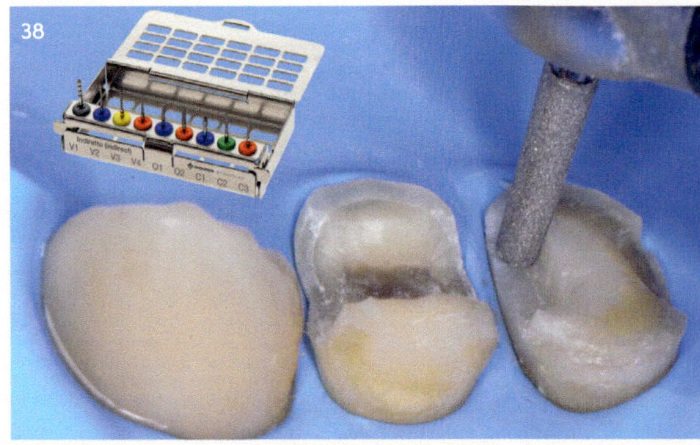

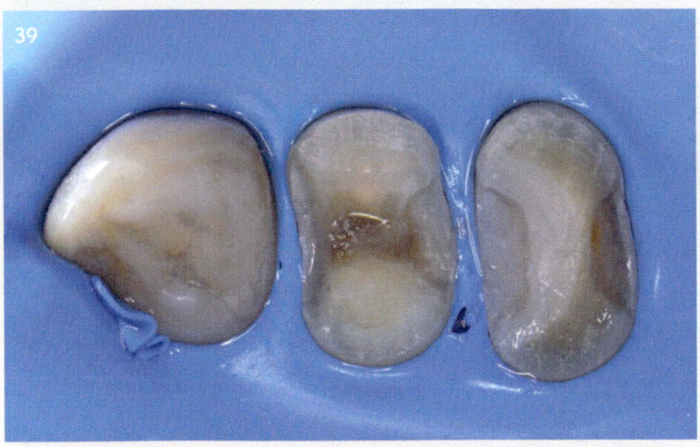

Figure 37 Reduction of the occlusal surface of the tooth by using the Style Indiretto Burs Kit (Intensiv, Switzerland).

Figure 38 Flat end bur for finishing the preparation (Style Indiretto Burs Kit – Intensiv, Switzerland).

Figure 39 Final preparation design under rubber dam. Cavities have detailed sharp margins, no undercuts, accessibility of subgingival margins, and no contact with adjacent teeth.

Figure 40 Final preparation before the final impression.

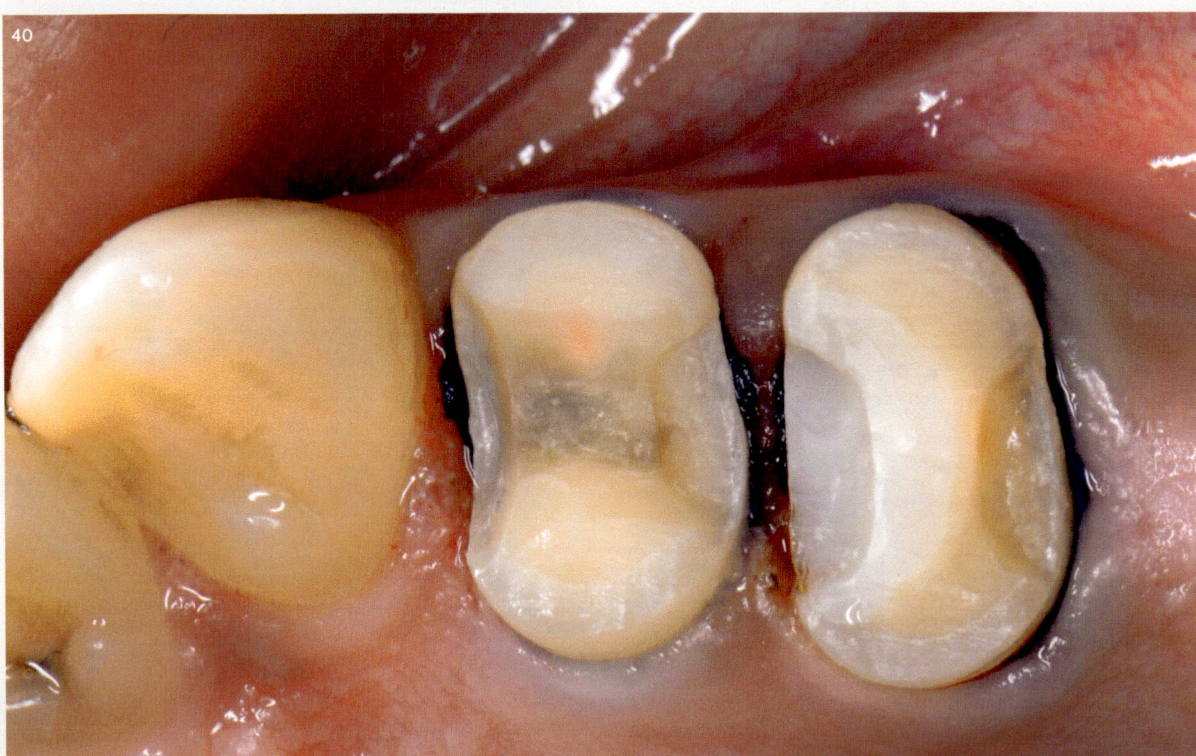

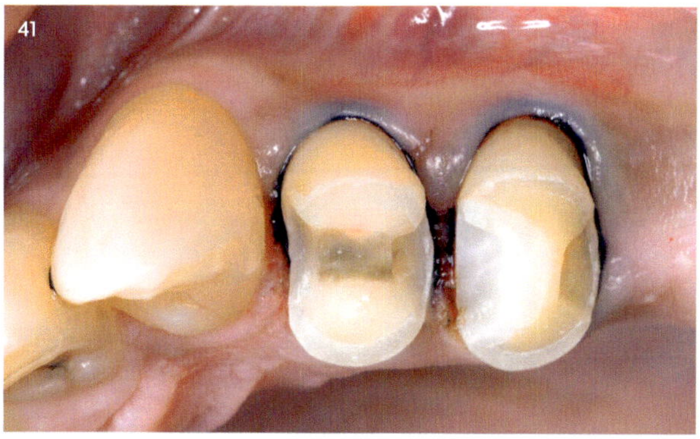

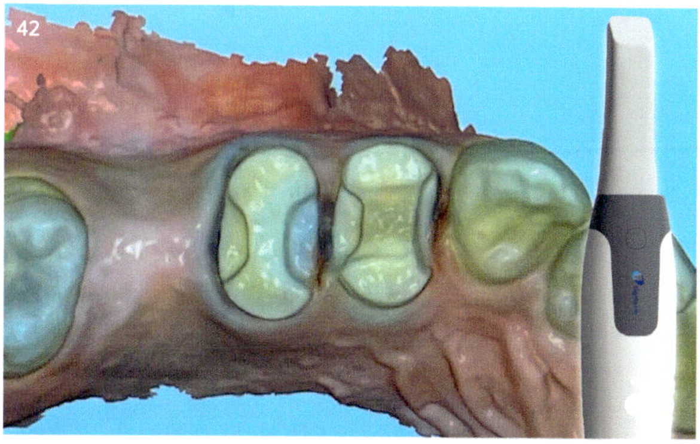

Figure 41 Final view of the teeth ready for the impression.

Figure 42 Final impression by intra-oral scanner (Helios 600 from Eighteeth, Changzhou, China).

Figure 43 Liquid dam: the material is ideal for provisionalizing non-retentive preparation as it is friendly to the soft tissue for up to 2–3 weeks.

Figure 44 A digital scan was taken; here you can see a screenshot from the standard tessellation language (STL) file and details of the preparation without the high definition.

Figure 45 A three-dimensional (3D) model showing the overlay project.

Figure 46 Lithium disilicate pressed overlay veneer (IPS e.max Press).

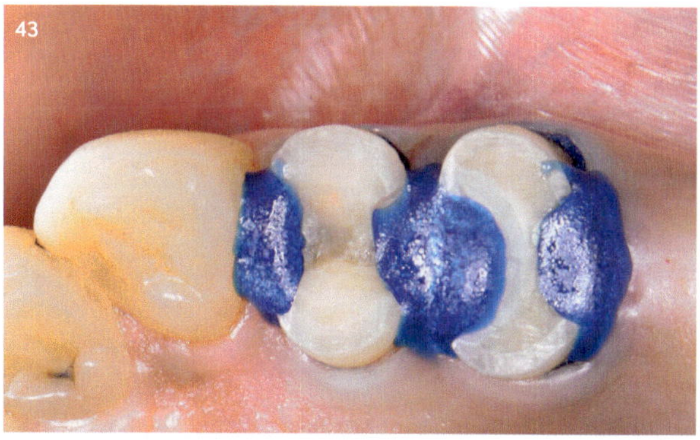

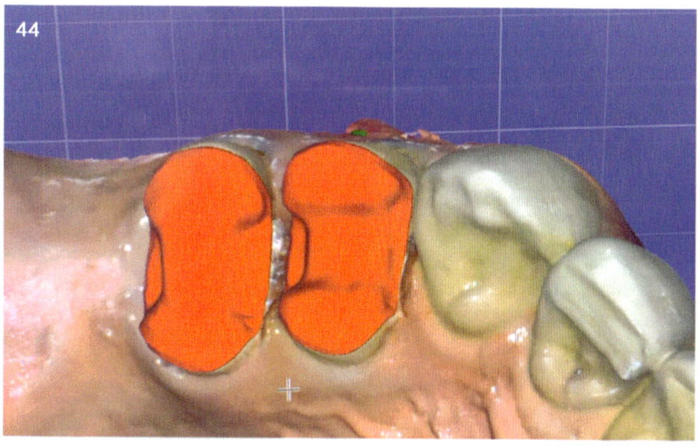

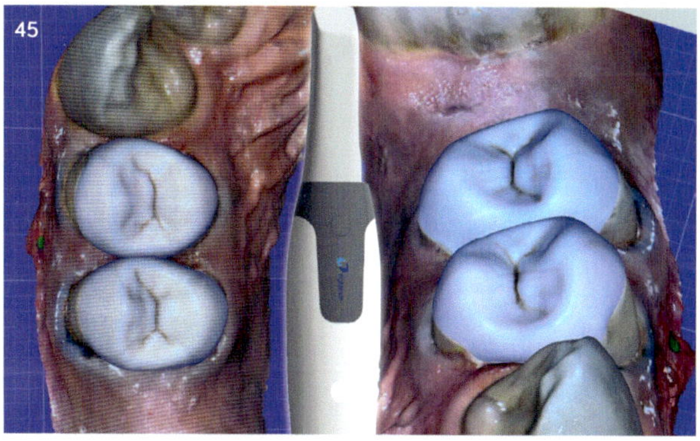

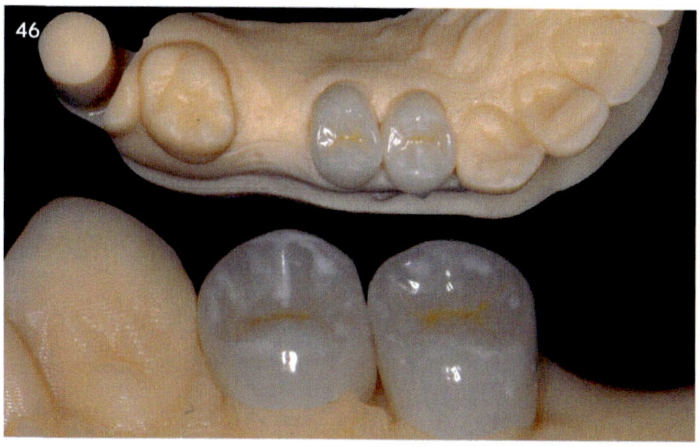

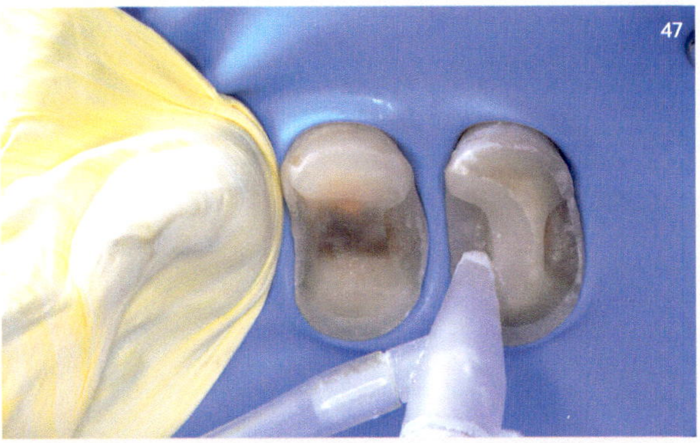

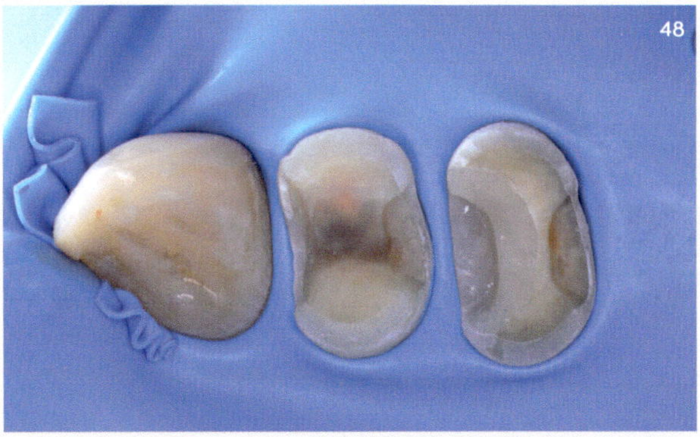

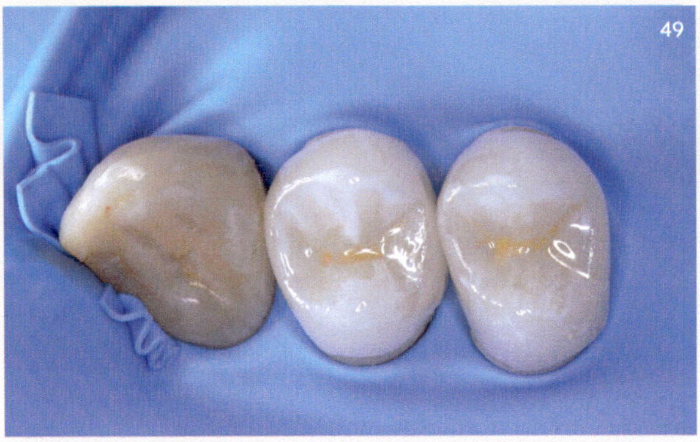

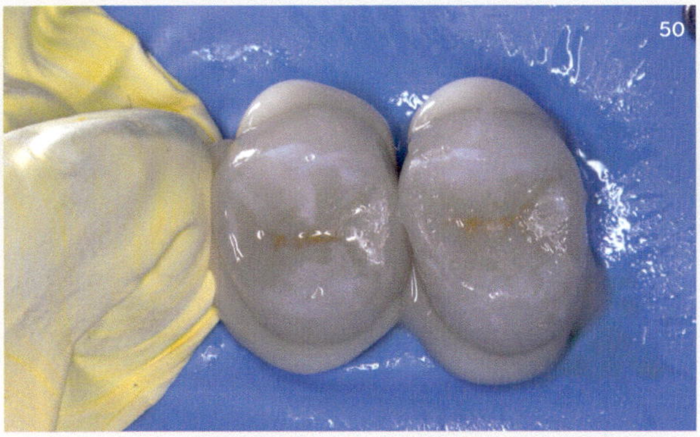

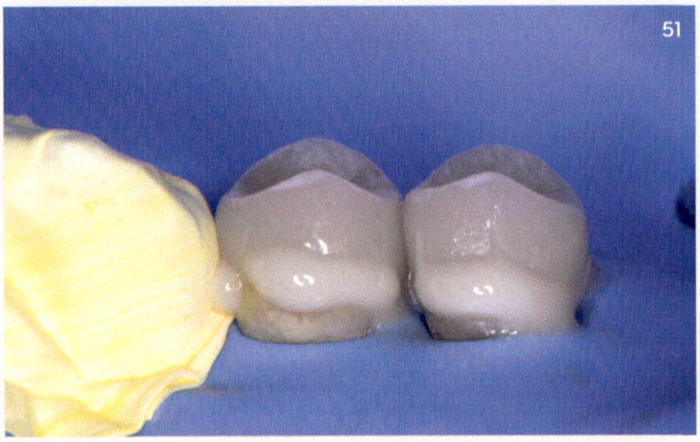

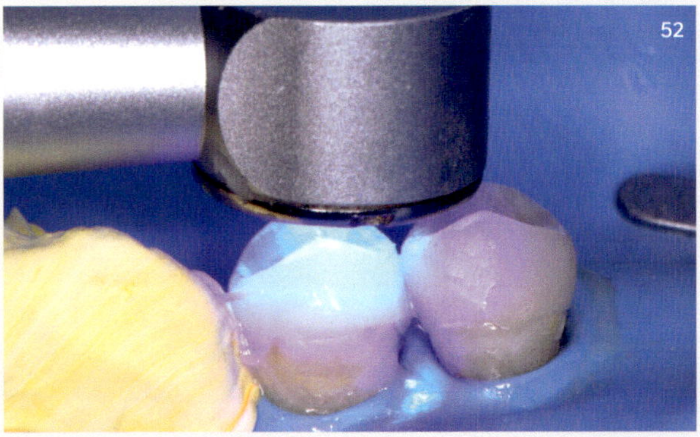

Figure 47 Using aluminum oxide 53-micron particles in order to clean and reactivate the tooth structure and composite before the cementation.

Figure 48 After sandblasting teeth were perfectly clean and ready for the bonding procedures.

Figure 49 Try in was carried out under rubber dam isolation to check proximal and marginal fit.

Figure 50 Resin cement was used for cementation.

Figure 51 Buccal view of resin cement was used for cementation.

Figure 52 A multi-wave curing pen (Curing Pen, Eighteeth, Changzhou, China) was used during cementation.

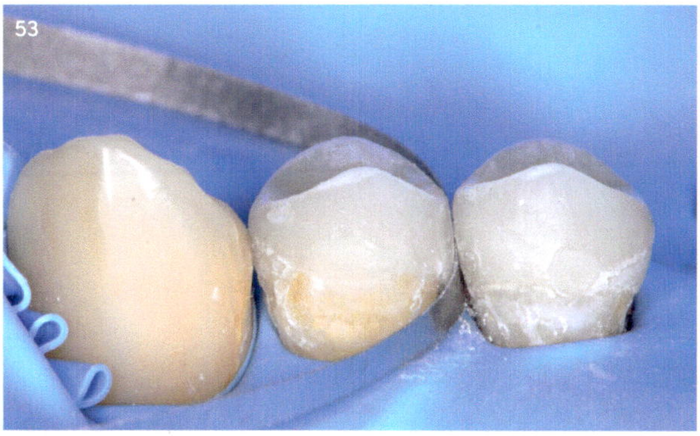

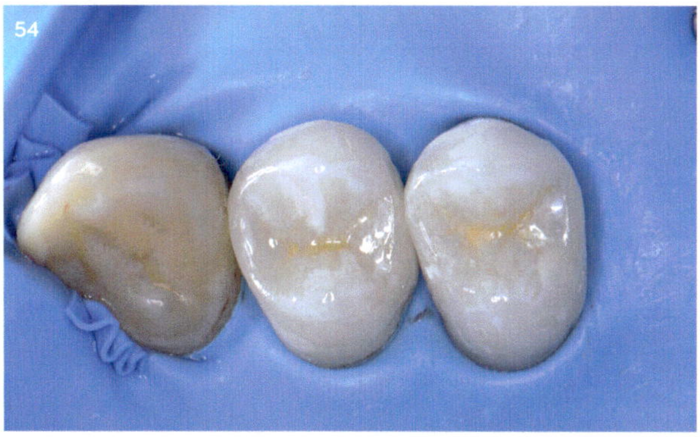

Figure 53 Finishing the inter-dental area by using metal strip (one side cutting).

Figure 54 Painted lithium disilicate (IPS e.max Press, Ivoclar Vivadent) overlay after adhesive cementation in isolated field with rubber dam.

Figure 55 Restoration in oral cavity with excellent morphological functional and esthetic integration.

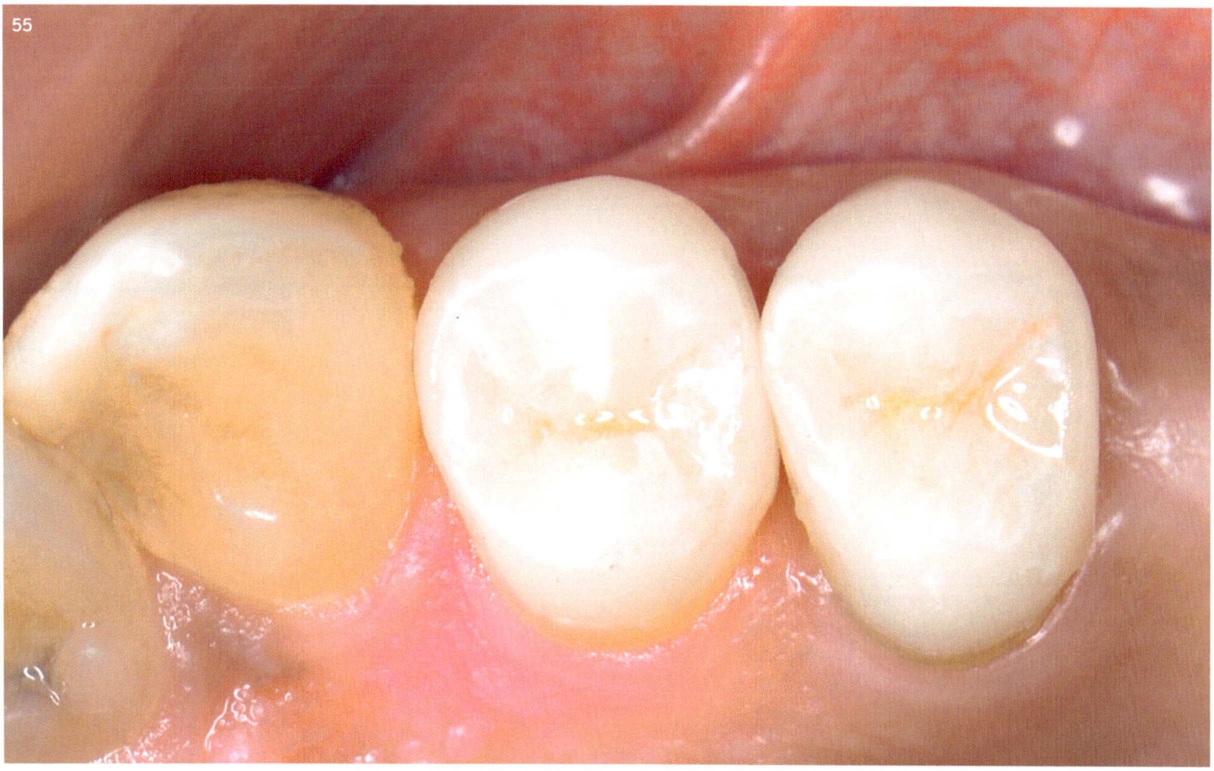

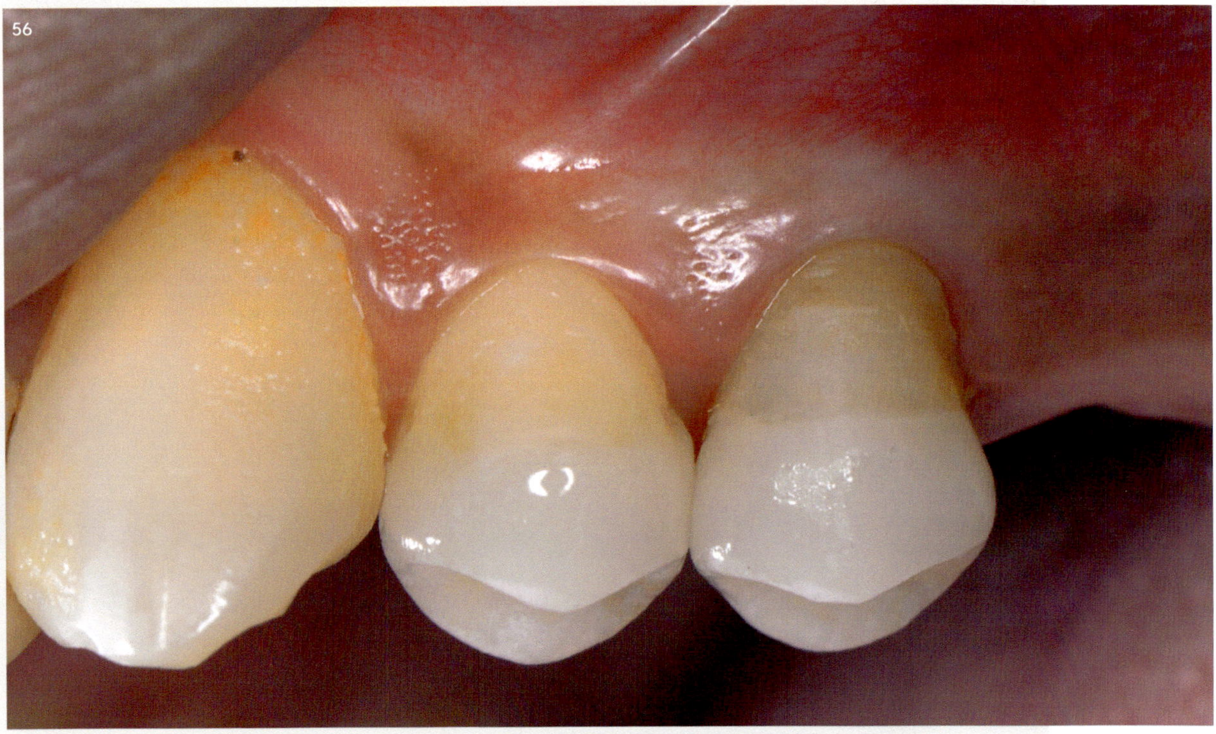

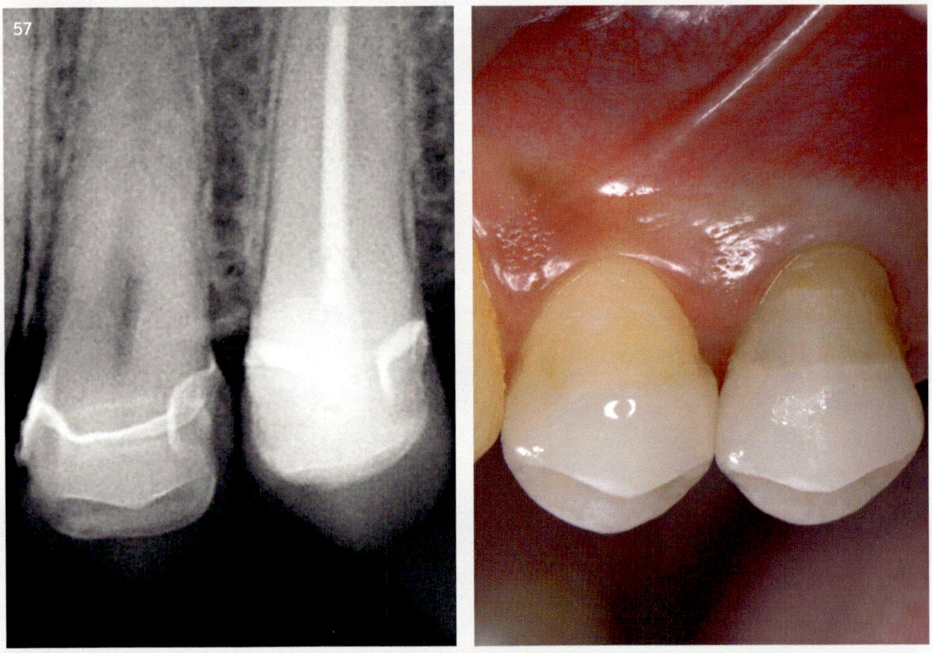

Figure 56 The indirect composite restoration after adhesive cementation with good esthetic, morphological, and functional integration.

Figure 57 Final situation and X-ray.

CONCLUSIONS

Modern restorative dentistry is substantially adhesive. The conservative spirit should pervade all of the dental procedures. In addition, preserving healthy tissue has become the priority. With this approach, indirect adhesive restorations are indicated in large cavities associated with cuspal coverage and absent or reduced amounts of cervical enamel.

The cavity preparation techniques for indirect restorations are different from the principles used for metal restorations or crown preparation. They allow a more conservative and esthetic dentistry, and they are a prerequisite for good cavity sealing, less postoperative sensitivity, and less marginal discoloration that can lead to secondary caries.

BIBLIOGRAPHY

1. Frankenberger R, Petschelt A, Krämer N. Leucite-reinforced glass ceramic inlays and onlays after six years: Clinical behavior. *Oper Dent.* 2000;25(6):459–465.
2. Reis B, Walther W. Clinical long-term results and 10-year Kaplan-Meier estimation of computer-aided machined CEREC restorations. *Int J Comput Dent.* 2000;3(1):9-23.
3. Reich SM, Wichmann M, Rinne H, Shortall A. Clinical performance of large, all-ceramic CAD/CAM-generated restorations after three years: A pilot study. *J Am Dent Assoc.* 2004;135(5):605–612.
4. Beier US, Kapferer I, Dumfahrt H. Clinical long-term evaluation and failure characterization of all-ceramic restoration. *Int J Prosthodont.* 2012;25(1):70–8.
5. Dietschi D, Spreafico R. Adhesive Metal-Free Restorations: Current Concepts for the Esthetic Treatment of Posterior Teeth. *Quintessence pub.* 1997.
6. Dietschi D, Magne P, Holz J. Recent trends in esthetic restorations for posterior teeth. *Quintessence Int.* 1994 Oct;25(10):659-677.
7. Signore A, Benedicenti S, Convani U, Ravera G. A 4–6 year retrospective clinical study of cracked teeth restored with bonded indirect resin composite onlays. *Int J Prosthodont.* 2007;20:609–616.
8. Magne P. Composite resins and bonded porcelain: the postamalgam era? *J Calif Dent Assoc.* 2006;34: 135–147.
9. Mehl A, Kunzelmann KH, Folwaczny M, Hickel R. Stabilization effects of CAD/CAM ceramic restorations in extended MOD cavities. *J Adhes Dent.* 2004;6:239–245.
10. Stappert CF, Abe P, Kurths V, Gerds T, Strub JR. Masticatory fatigue, fracture resistance, and marginal discrepancy of ceramic partial crowns with and without coverage of compro- mised cusps. *J Adhes Dent.* 2008;10:41–48.
11. Federlin M, Sipos C, Hiller KA, Thonemann B, Schmalz G. Partial ceramic crowns. Influence of preparation design and luting material on margin integrity–a scanning electron microscopic study. *Clin Oral Investig.* 2005;9:8–17.
12. Rocca GT, Krejci I. Crown and post-free adhesive restorations for endodontically treated posterior teeth: from direct composite to endocrowns. *Eur J Esthet Dent.* 2013;8:156–179.
13. Fennis WM, Kuijs RH, Kreulen CM, Verdonschot N, Creugers NH. Fatigue resistance of teeth restored with cuspal coverage composite restorations. *Int J Prosthodont.* 2004;17:313–317.
14. Stavridakis MM, Krejci I, Magne P. Immediate dentin sealing of onlay preparations: thickness of pre-cured dentin bonding agent and effect of surface cleaning. *Oper Dent.* 2005;30:747–757.
15. Magne P, Nielsen B. Interactions between impression materials and immediate dentin sealing. *J Prosthet Dent.* 2009;102:298–305.

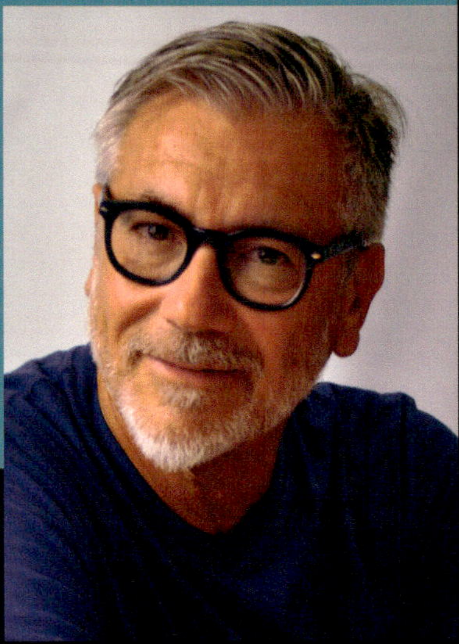

DANIELE RONDONI

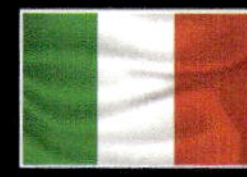

Italy

MDT Rondoni was born in Savona in 1961 where he lives and has worked in his own laboratory since 1982 with his collaborators.
He graduated from the dental technicians school IPSIA "P. Gaslini" in Genoa in 1979. He continued his education by attending relevant workshops for the "Italian dental school" and furthered his professional experience in Switzerland, Germany and Japan where he attended Master "Hitoshi Aoshima" training center, increasing knowledge regarding the porcelain layering and Internal Live Stain technique that him invented.
Particularly devoted to the morphology and dental aesthetics, MDT Rondoni has collaborated in the development of aesthetic dental restoration materials and is author of *Techniques of Ceramic multistratification* (ed. UTET) where examined in depth the metal framework treatment and porcelain layering technique.
He has created a manual for laboratory work on the use of composite materials by determining work protocols for the indirect technique and also for the technique of pressing composite structures on metal, known as the "inverse stratification system" which he designed.
MDT Rondoni is the author of numerous articles on aesthetic restoration published in Italy and abroad. Some of his cases are published in the text by Vanini L, Mangani F, and Klimovscaja O. *The Conservative Restoration of Anterior Teeth.* 2nd ed. (ACME Viterbo; 2007). Other clinical cases are presented in *Restorative Dentistry: Treatment procedures and future prospects* (ed. E Masson).
He contributed with dedicated chapters, regarding the colour evolution in dentistry in *Layer 1* and *Layer 2* books by Manauta, Salat, Devoto, Putignano (Quintessence pub.).
He puts special attention to technology from start to work with a digital approach and contribution to the research and evolution of new aesthetic generation materials dedicated as Composite and Zirconia, topic of his education activity and lectures in several congress in the world.
MDT Rondoni is an active member of the European Academy of Esthetic Dentistry (EAED), active member and speaker of the Italian Society of Ceramic Esthetic Dentistry (SICED), active member of the Italian Aesthetic Dentistry (IAED), Honorary member of StyleItaliano.
MDT Rondoni is a teacher and trainer in practical Master for Digital and Aesthetic dentistry at the graduate school of Turin, Brescia, Roma, Chieti (Italy).

DIGITAL DENTAL COLOR, PRACTICAL APPLICATIONS WITH STATE-OF-THE-ART COLORIMETERS

DANIELE RONDONI, MDT
ROSSI ROBERTO, CDT

In its vast complexity, color science embraces physics, mathematics, geometry, measurements, perception, chemistry, optics, art, and human psychology. All in all, color is psychophysics in a nutshell.

As the final restoration has to be perfect to the eye of the clinical technician and patient, dental color assessment requires extreme precision, computing, and execution. This task can be carried out digitally or analogically.

For obvious reasons, eyeball-metrics is the most commonly used method among clinicians[1]. Despite being the most widespread method, due to its lack of objectivity, it is also the least appreciated within the scientific community and yet, the eye remains the final judge, regardless of the color method selected or used.

After all, what matters the most is the look of the final restoration when fitted in the mouth. This is what makes determination of a dental shade extremely important, regardless of the color matching method used.

Despite having been available for over 30 years, digital color assessment methods have become popular only lately, as they are becoming more common both in clinics and in labs.

DISCUSSION AND CLINICAL CASE

Dental shade guides

Stock shade guides have long been the first resource for dental color determination; they have been improved over time with Vita Classical as the benchmark for the gold standard.

Common homemade strategies have been proposed throughout the years in order to optimize the use of stock shade guides[2]. Incrementation of pink composite gives the shade guide a better context as it makes human perception slightly better. Pink pastes make the tooth look more realistic, as if it were coming out from the gum (1). Although this does not solve the core issue of stock shade guides, it slightly helps focusing the attention on the full tooth. Commercial pink shade guide holders by different brands have been proposed to this end, yet they may be easily fabricated with acrylic resin by any clinician.

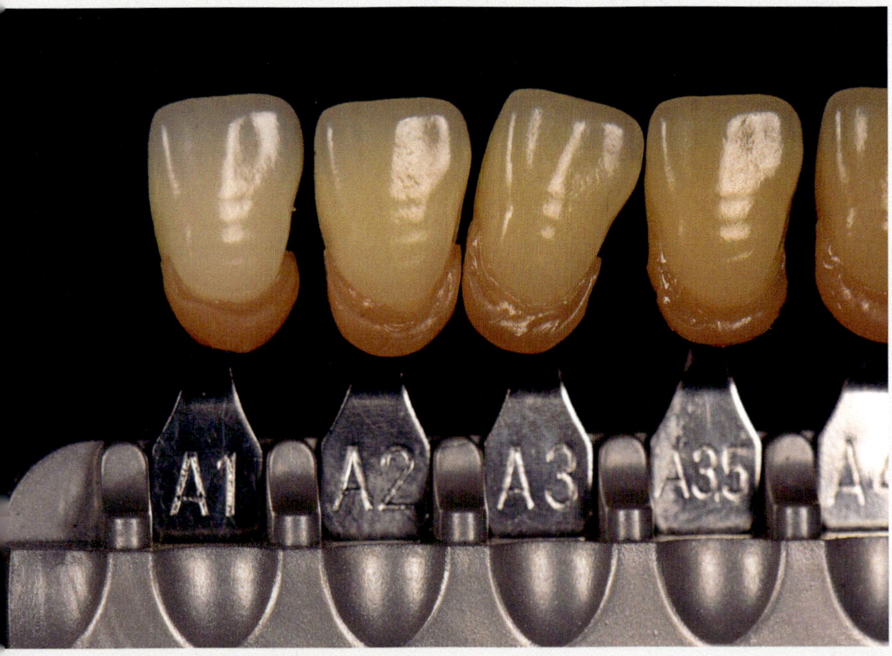

Figure 1 Vita Classical shade guide with a pink add-on to improve its context and increasing its efficiency in color matching. One of the many hacks proposed during the years, it had limited success.

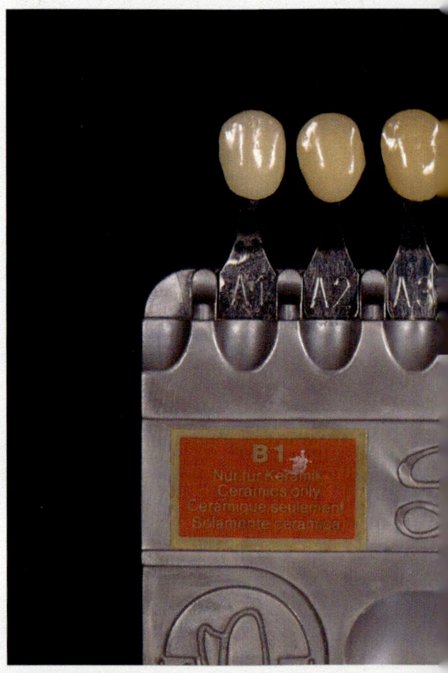

Figure 2 Vita Classical shade guide with the cervical and incisal portion trimmed. This was proposed to increase color matching precision. Other of the many hacks proposed, it not only had limited success, but it was the origin of other problems.

Another DIY method aiming at optimizing stock shade guides is by trimming the cervical and incisal portions (2), leaving the area where the color is more even throughout the surface. This eliminates all forms of distractions, as for many people, the translucent mass in the incisal area and the dimmer cervical area are a disturbance rather than an aid. This area-trimming technique makes the shade guide look more like a solid color[3]. Needless to say, this comes with a price as the useful area of color reference, which is the center of the shade guide, decreases importantly. A ready-made solution is the Vita Color-guide, which is made without the incisal and the cervical areas.

Personalized shade guides are easy to self-manufacture, with the same materials from the actual intra-oral restoration[4]. Initially, they were proposed as the ultimate solution, at least at a theoretical level, but soon big problems were found as they did not perfectly match the color of the stock shade guide or showed several discrepancies with the final restorations (3).

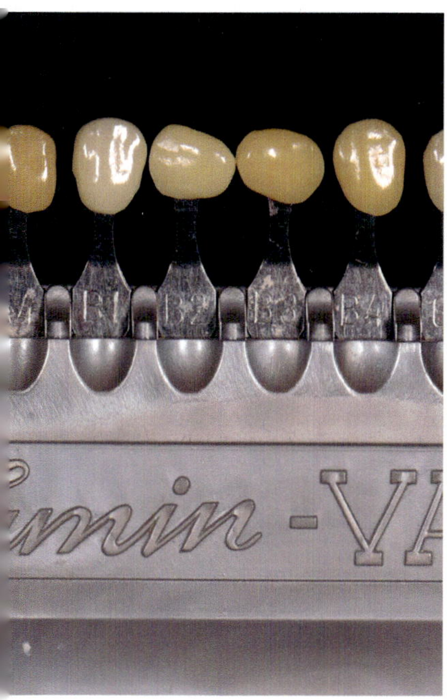

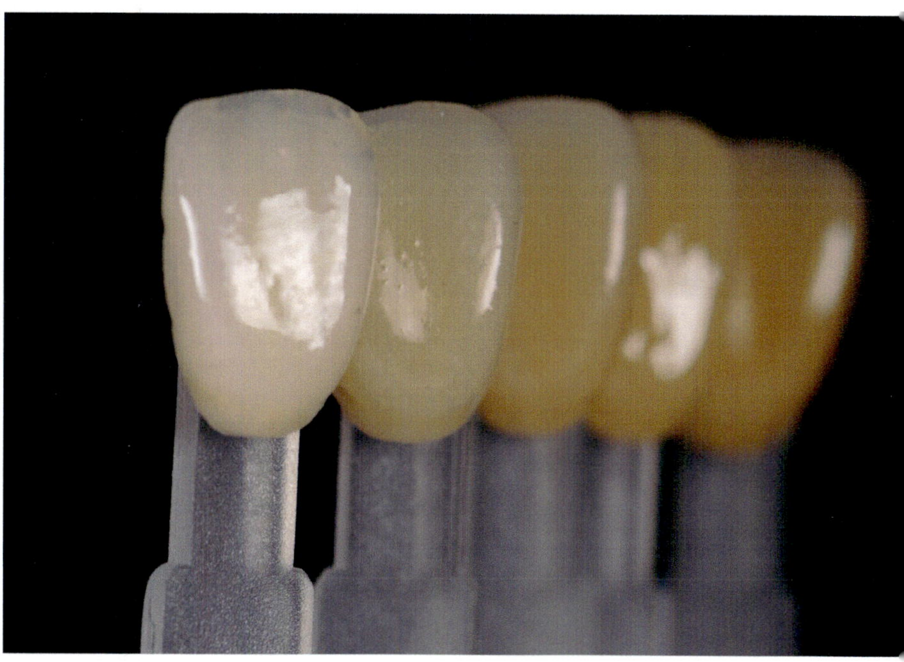

Figure 3 2-layers personalized shade guide. These make composite layering more predictable, but still add limits and invisible problems.

Optishade-StyleItaliano

Optishade StyleItaliano (Smile Line, Switzerland) is a digital colorimeter, specifically designed for its dental application that functions with Apple smart devices (iPhone and iPad). Its color measurement high precision (DE94 0,2-0,4) and accuracy, and L*a*b* and L*C*h reading, allow for real-time cross-check data with several pre-loaded shade guide databases such as Vita Classical, Vita 3D master (📷 4).

When we have an accurate and reliable method for color matching, when measuring the same subject we should obtain the same numerical values[5]. Our task consists in repeating the same scenario in every measurement, so color should be measured with the following setting:

- Using a device that has a minimal discrepancy with its own measures (intra device precision)
- Using a device that has a minimal discrepancy with other devices of its kind (inter device precision)
- Same background
- Same centering and positioning
- Clean teeth
- No external light contamination
- Hydrated teeth

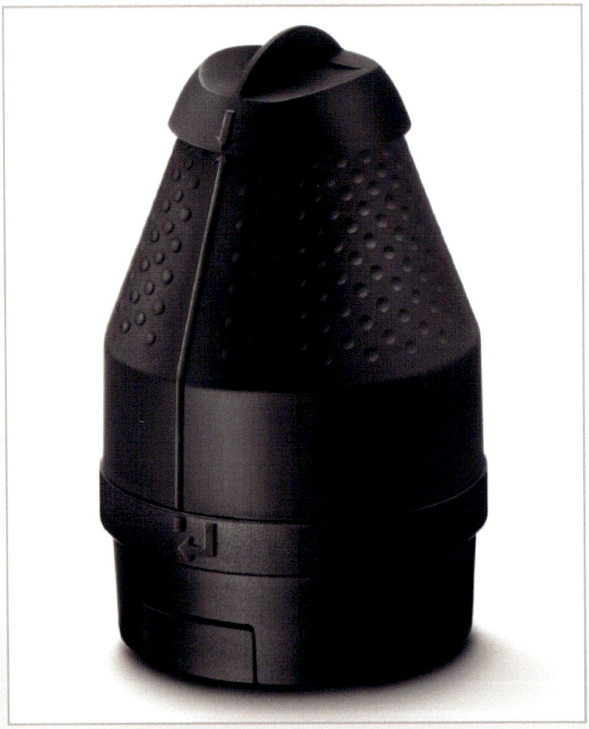

Figure 4 Color matching by replicating the same scenario.

With control of these simple parameters it is possible to accurately reproduce the scenario and have a reliable color measurement.
Positioning is the main parameter to obtain reputable and reliable measurements. If the device perceives an error, the technician will replicate it.
Perception in dentistry is incredibly complex, but our final aim is, once fitted into the mouth, being positively judged by our and patient's eyes.
It is the good appearance in the mouth that counts, and the digital technology is here to make this happens easier, faster and in a more predictable way. The shade guide of the future needs to be able to tell us the color in an understandable way!
This is the reason why our workflow has evolved towards reliability; where the technician and the clinician can trust one measurement and deliver a perfect restoration, without having to see the patient, and with no shade guides or repetitions.

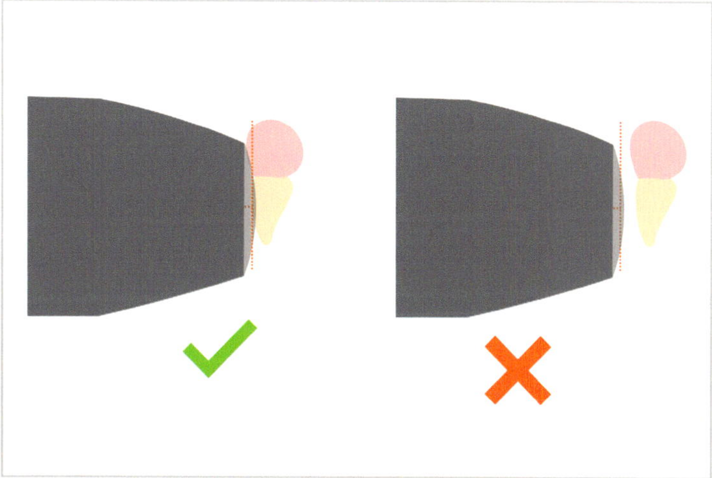

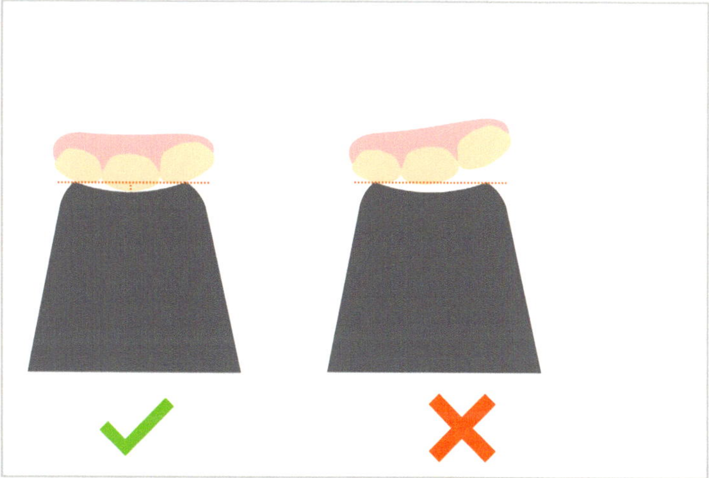

Clinical application

Single central crown over implant

In the following clinical case, a single central was restored and the color was estimated and performed with the aid of a digital colorimeter (Optishade).

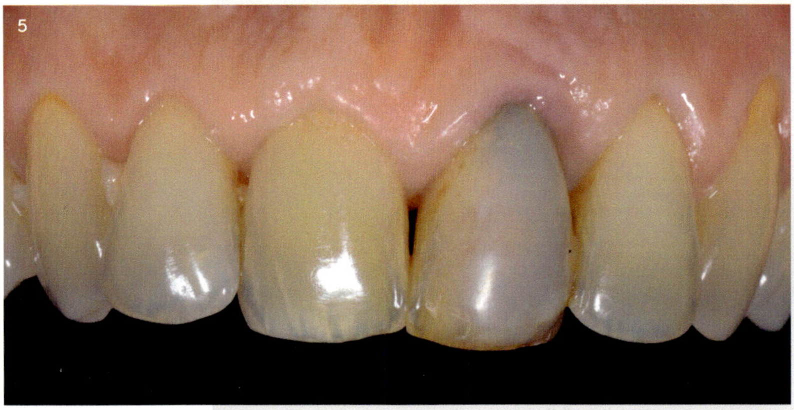

Figure 5 Initial situation: fractured tooth was programmed for atraumatic extraction and immediate implant.

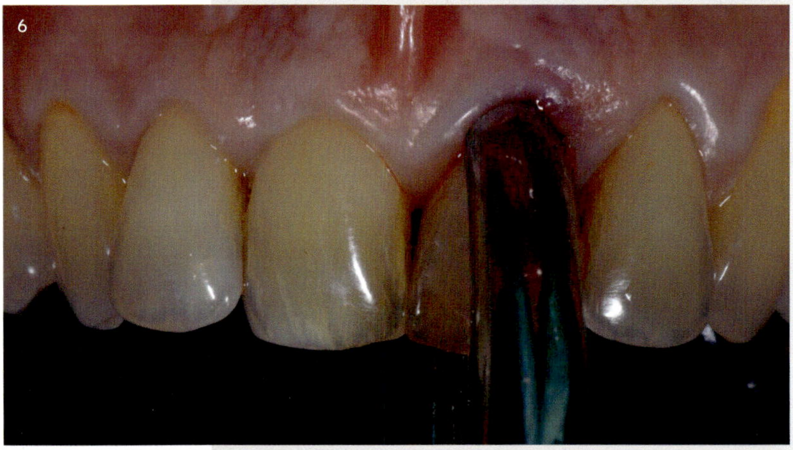

Figure 6 The tooth was extracted.

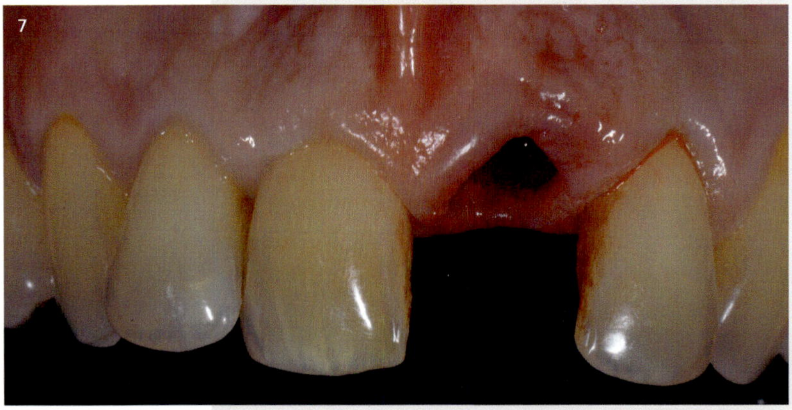

Figure 7 In the same appointment, the implant was placed.

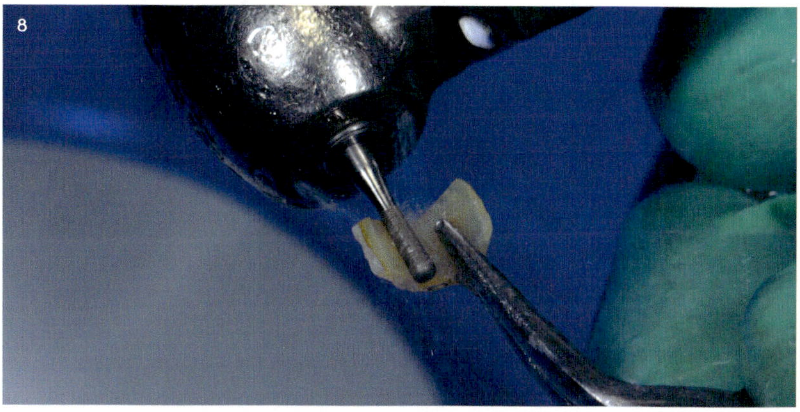

Figure 8 A tooth slice was prepared in order to preserve the buccal bone plate.

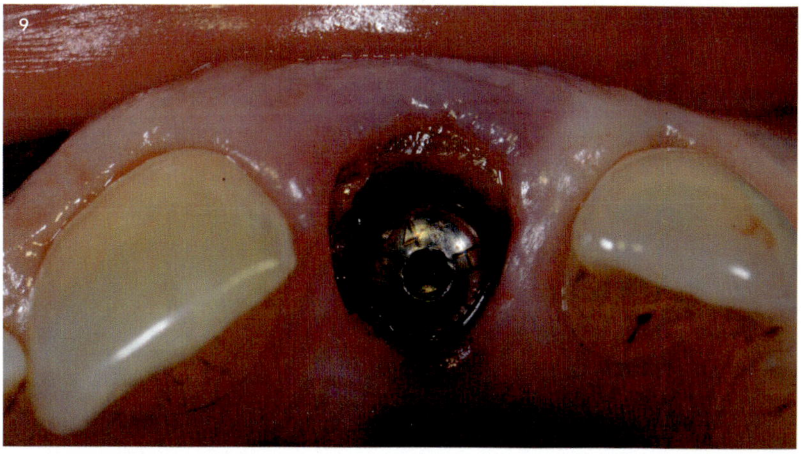

Figure 9 A shield technique was used to avoid the buccal plate collapse.

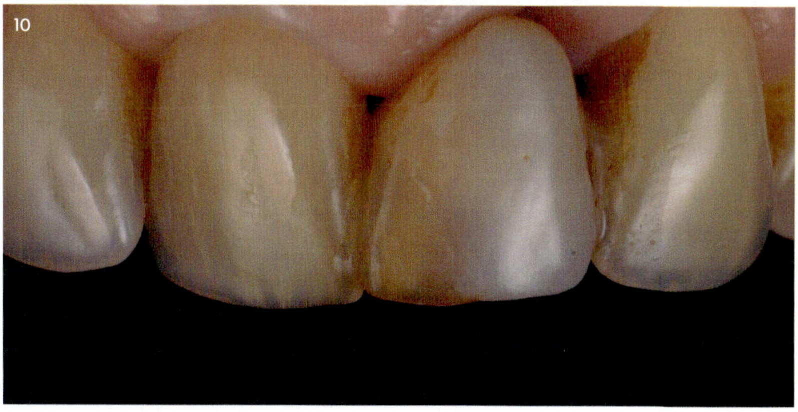

Figure 10 After 2 weeks it can be seen the healing of the socket under the temporary tooth bonded to the neighbor teeth.

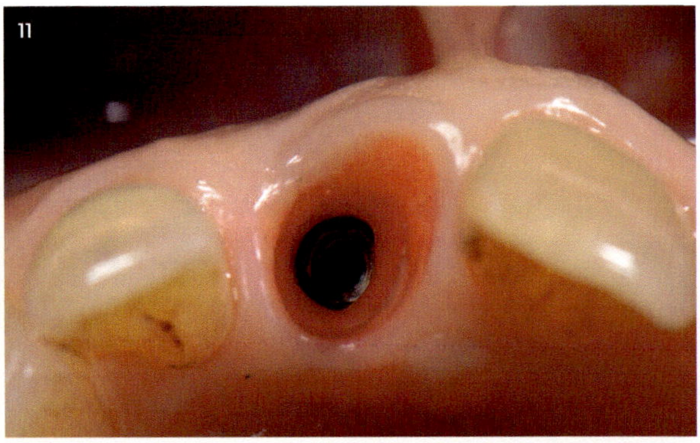

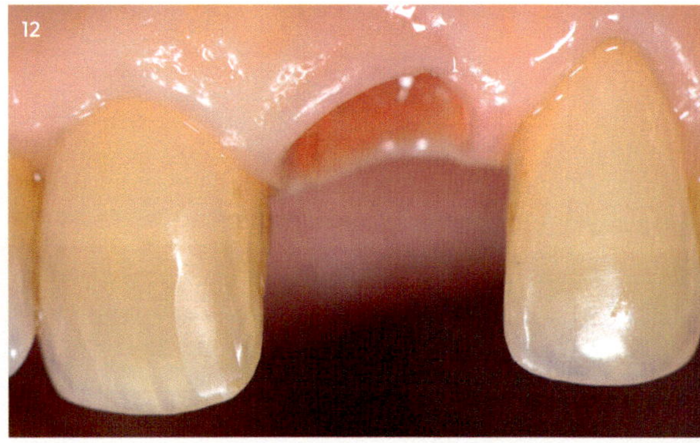

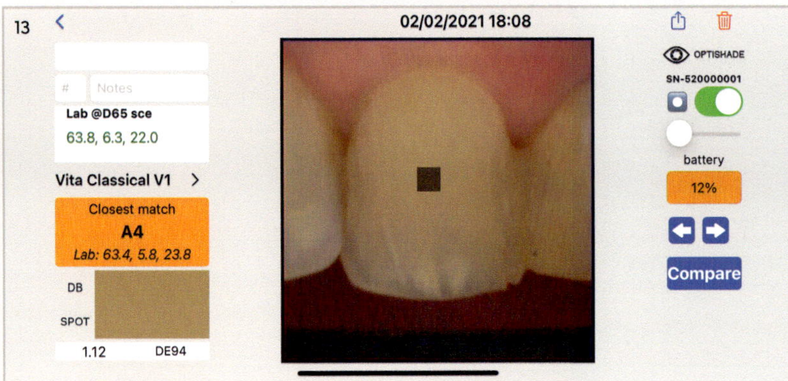

Figure 11 Frontal aspect of the site to be restored.

Figure 12 The healed peri-implant site ready for impression.

Figure 13 Target color is measured starting from the healthy tooth with Optishade. This information will be shared with the technician.

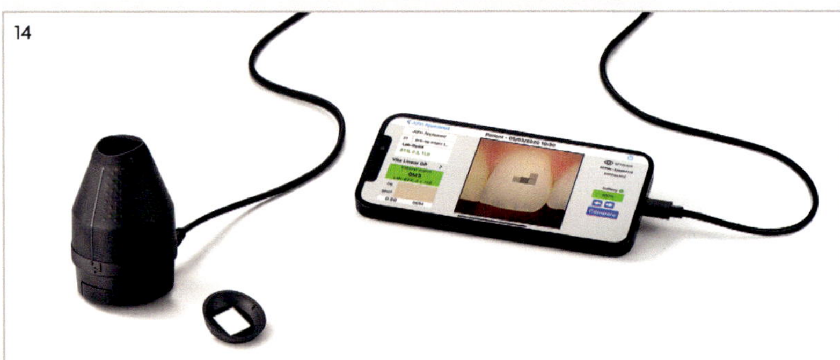

Figure 14 The measurement must be perfect following the aforementioned guidelines in order to minimize the risk of mistakes.

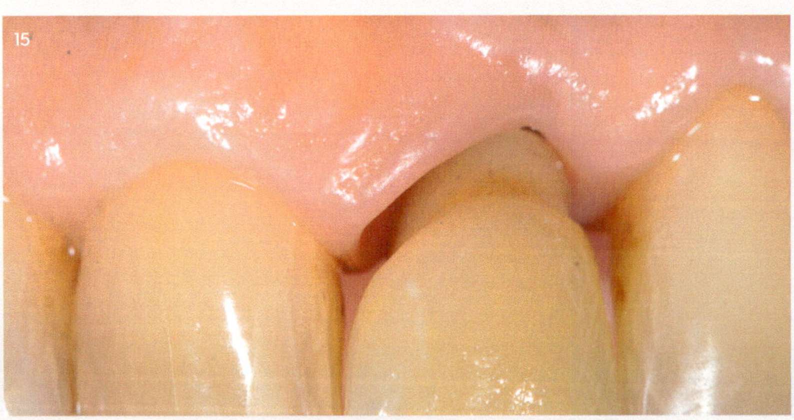

Figure 15 Try-in of the monolithic painted crown.

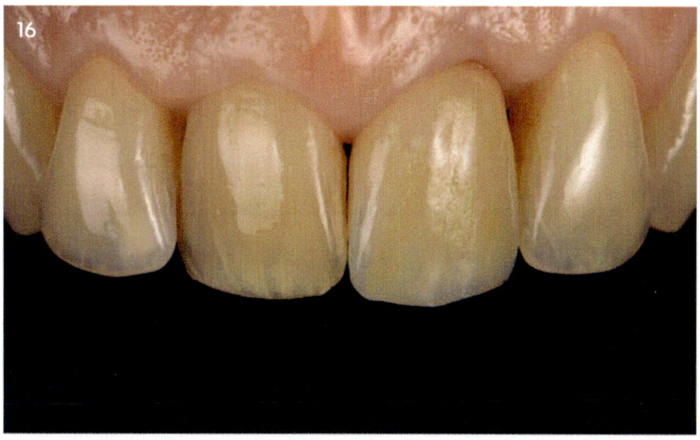

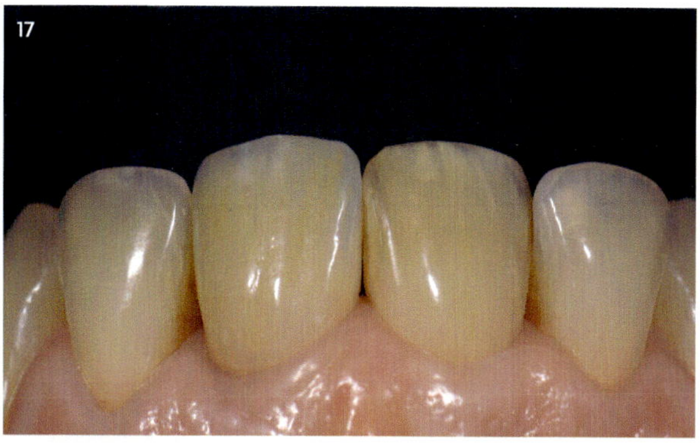

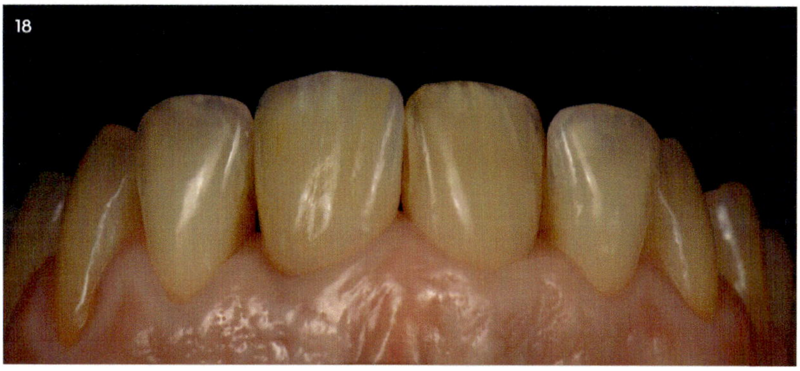

Figure 16 The try-in stage was successful, and no further corrections were needed.

Figure 17 1-year control shows a perfect integration.

Figure 18 Same control but with diffuse light to highlight the texture and shape.

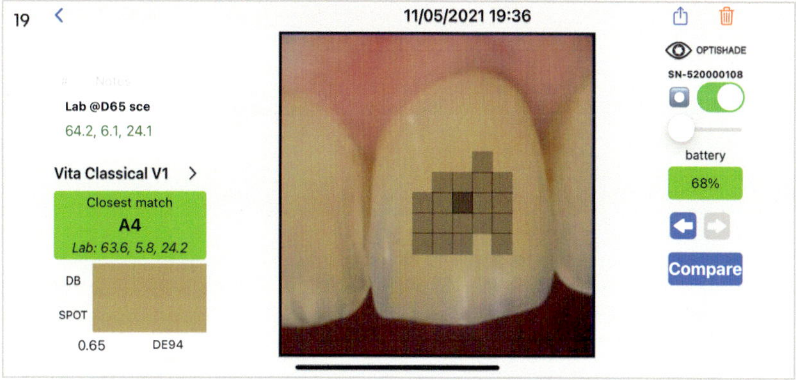

Figure 19 Resulting color from the crown manufactured in the laboratory, which gets very close to the color of the desired tooth.

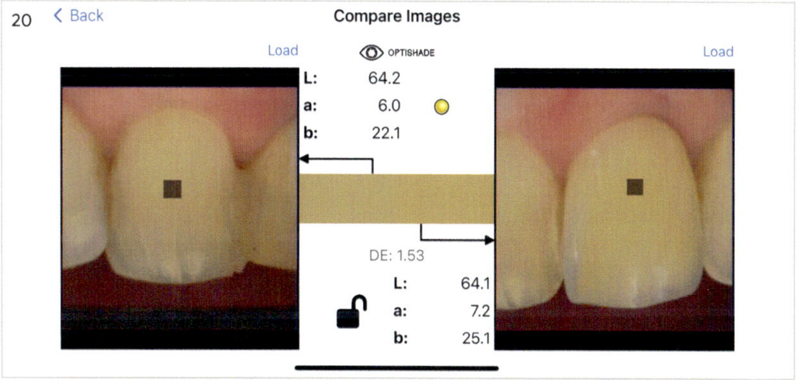

Figure 20 Direct comparison, gives a good match (good match is under 1.60 DE).

Where should we measure color

One of the hardest challenges in the dental color world is the integration of anterior restorations. This has been demonstrated to be very reliable when done with precise mathematical computation, particularly with ceramic mixing and layering.

For the best outcome of the mixing and layering ceramic software, the use of a high precision color matching device is mandatory. Optishade has proved to be the best for this use.

2 perfect color measurements must be provided:

- **A.** Target color: the desired color, the final goal. It is calculated from the adjacent healthy teeth or the closest good-looking restorations.
- **B.** Substrate: the color of the preparation where we will cement the restoration. It has the ability to modify the final color of the restoration and must be considered for the final calculation. Once all this information has been gathered, it is possible to calculate a multiple layered restoration which, alongside the stump, will generate the final color. With this raw restoration, which might even look odd outside its context, it will be possible to modify the unfavorable substrate so as to make the whole look as similar as possible or even identical to the desired color.
- **C.** Modifier: it has different aspect from the desired color as it is out-of-context and is not influenced by the substrate. Oftentimes, its aspect outside the restoration site is not good. The raw restoration is calculated mathematically in order to have the right layers and opacities to balance the chromatic change that will occur when the restoration and substrate are integrated, for this reason it is named "modifier".
- **D.** Final color: this is the result of the restoration and the substrate together within the mouth context; it happens when the restoration is in place with the final cement or with a try-in agent.

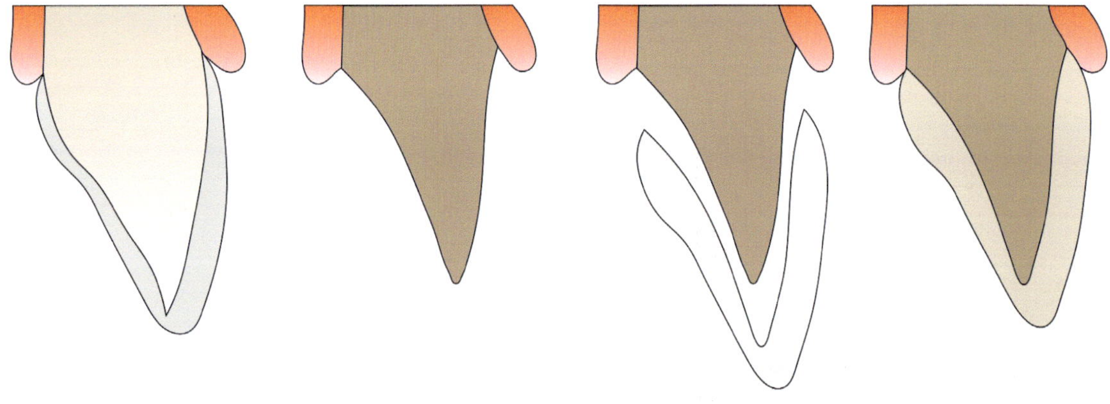

A Target color | B Substrate | C Modifier | D Final color: Modifier + substrate

Figures 21–22–23 When providing the target color and the substrate (in the case of an implant, there is not a substrate), the mixing software is able to predict the framework and the stratification to match the desired color.

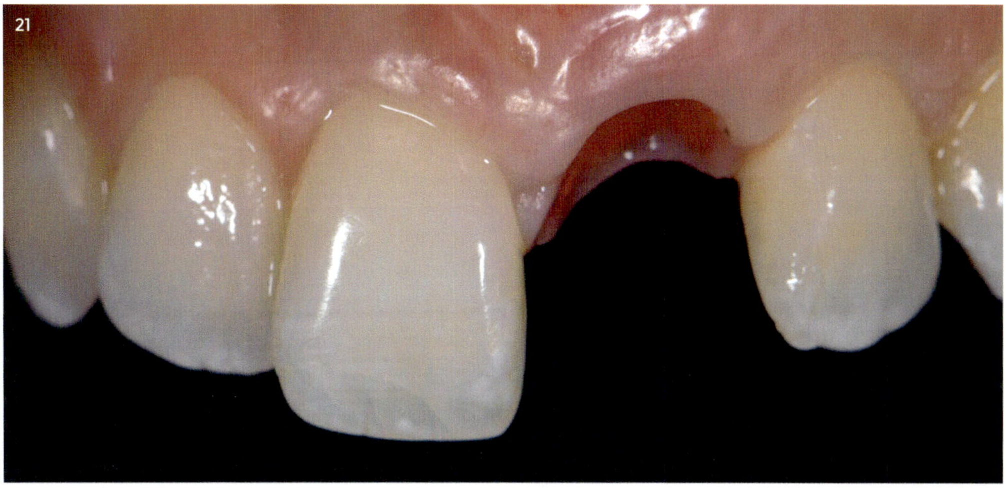

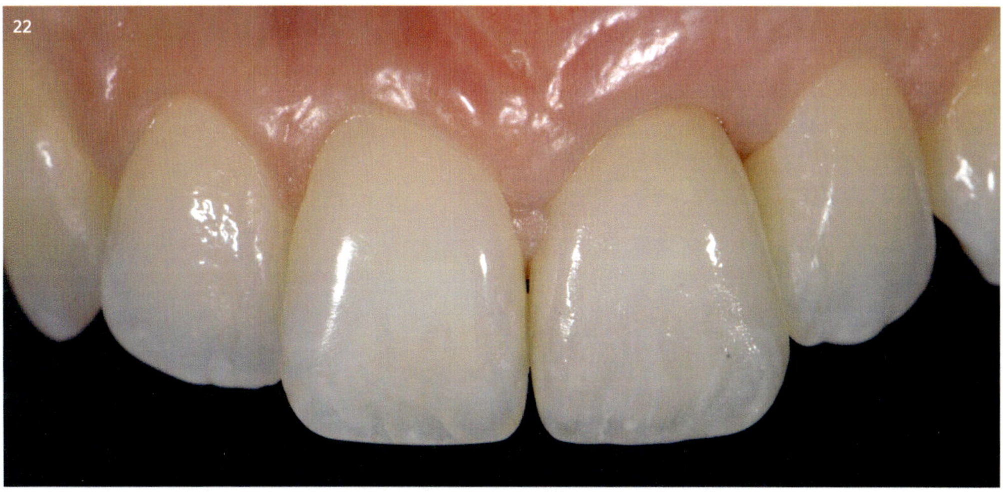

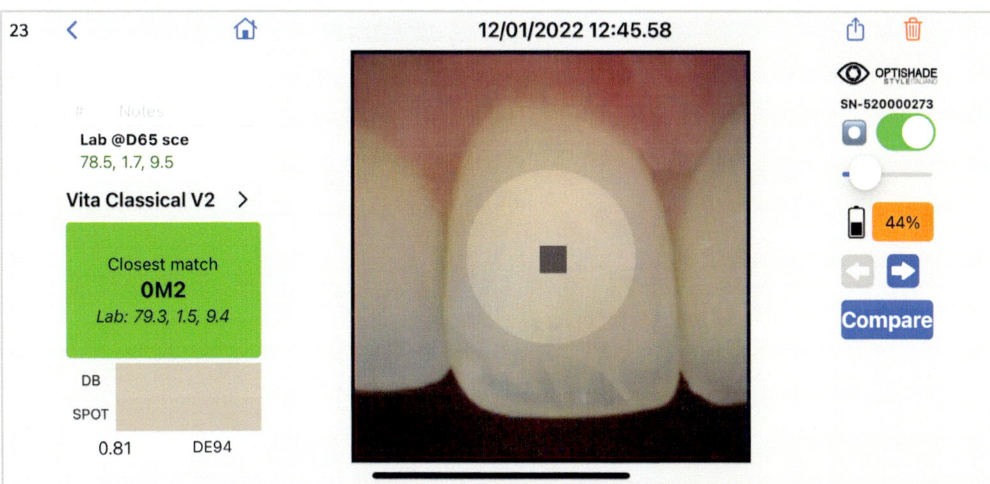

cont'd

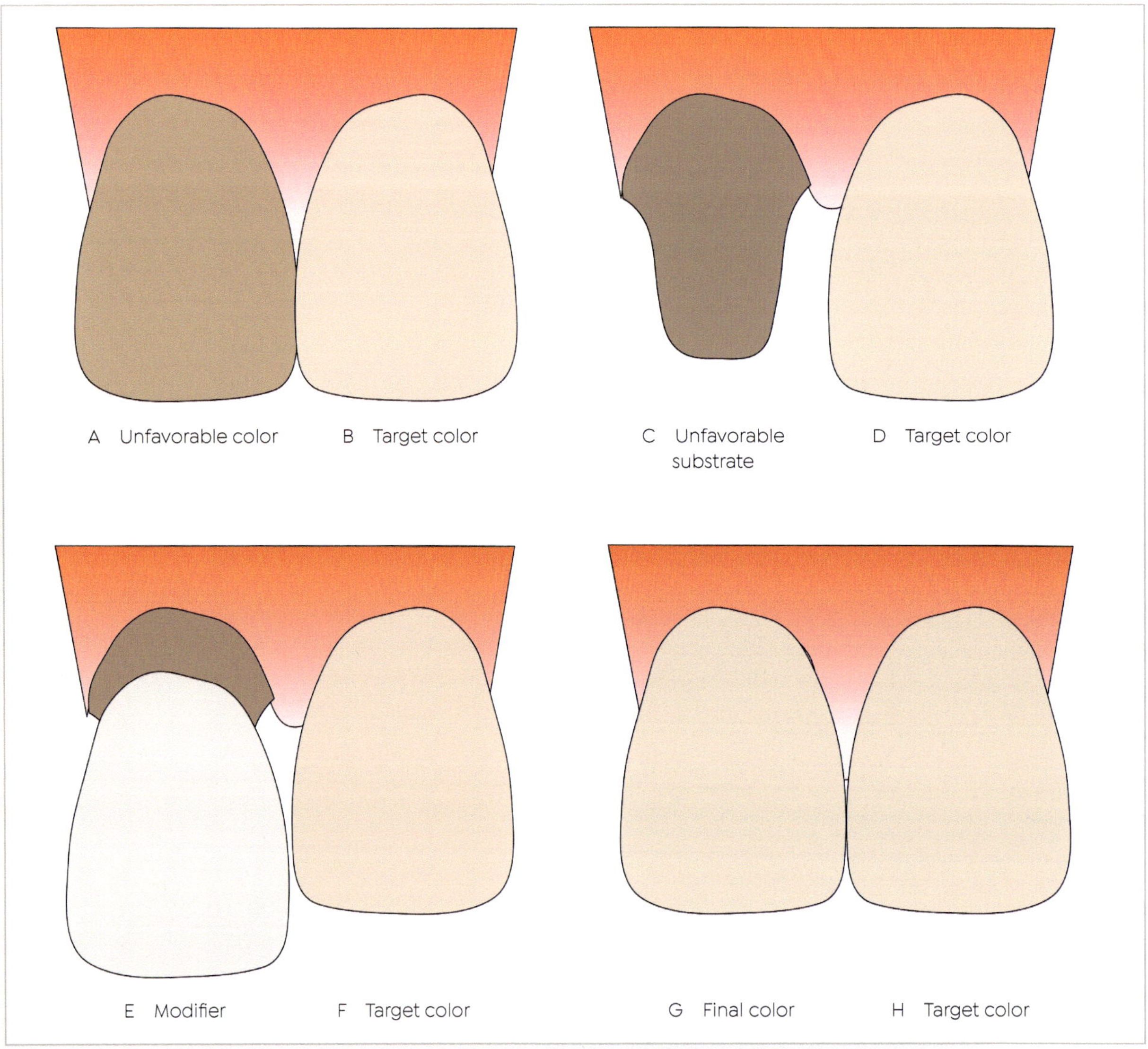

ΔE_{94}	Perception in the dental field
0	Identical perceived colors
< 0,67	Excellent match
0,67 to 1	Very good match
1 to 1,6	Good match
1,6 to 2,7	Acceptable mismatch
2,7 to 4,7	Evident mismatch
> 4,7	Unacceptable mismatch

The integrated restoration must give as a final result the desired color, or at least be very close to it. Restorations before integration and in-context try-in have a different appearance from the desired color.

Clinical application, central pairs with different substrates

In the following clinical case, two central incisors were restored and the color was assessed and achieved with the aid of a digital colorimeter (Optishade).

In a case where two centrals need to be restored, an undesirable problem that can be found is when the substrate of one or more have a non-favorable color. In the following case, calculations are made by specialized software (Matisse) and each of the monolithic substructures will have a different color but they will look the same once integrated into the substrate.

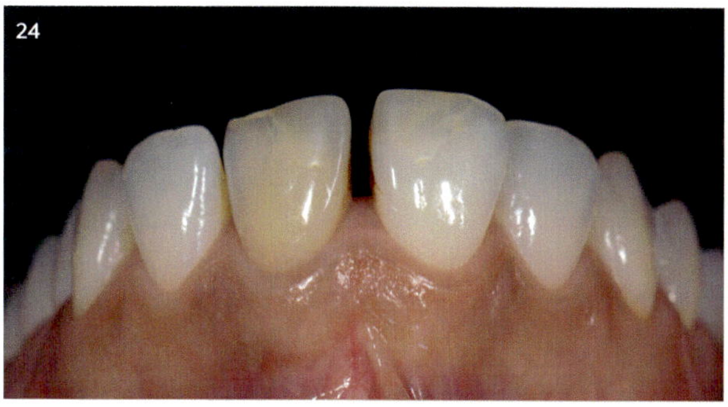

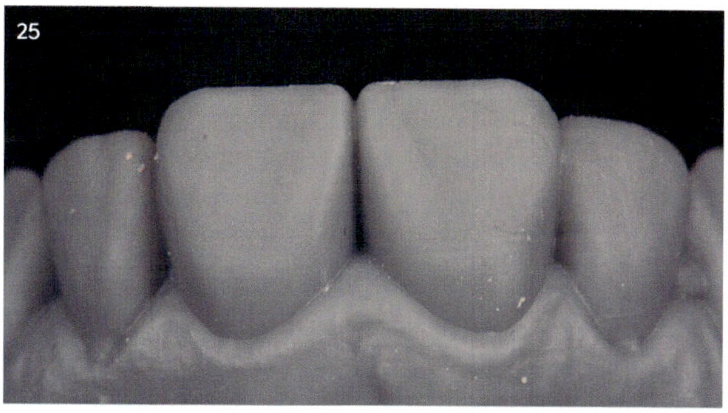

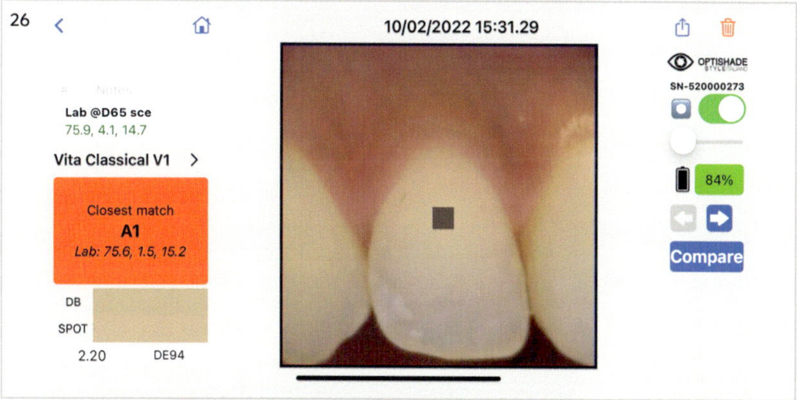

Figure 24 Initial situation, two chromatically and morphologically compromised teeth.

Figure 25 An additional wax-up was done, and a project for the final shape was proposed. From these shapes, the full treatment was then executed.

Figure 26 First of all, the target color is determined. It is done by measuring the most appealing color in the arch. In this case it's from the upper right lateral, which will set the color coordinates to be replicated in the ceramic restorations.

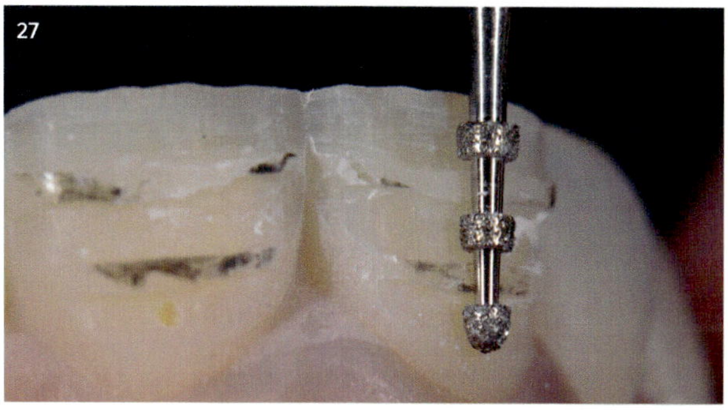

Figure 27 The teeth preparations were done over the mock-up. Calibrated burs were used over the resin, very little tooth was touched.

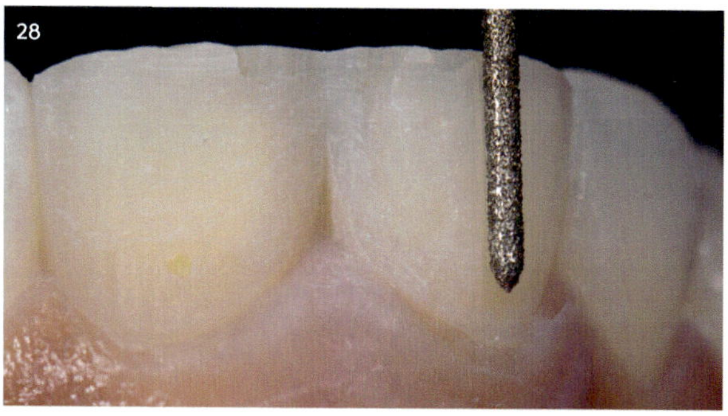

Figure 28 The final thickness was achieved by cancelling the depth marks. Almost no-prep was obtained.

Figures 29–30 Thickness obtained with preparation was exactly as expected from the wax-up.

Figure 31 Retraction cords were inserted with a special tweezer (Pick-pack) for the final impression.

Figures 32–33–34 Two disilicate veneers were milled in a 5-axis milling machine. Veneer from tooth 21 was BL1 and Veneer from the 11 was A1. Both veneers were synthesized and stained according to the numerical difference displayed with Optishade.

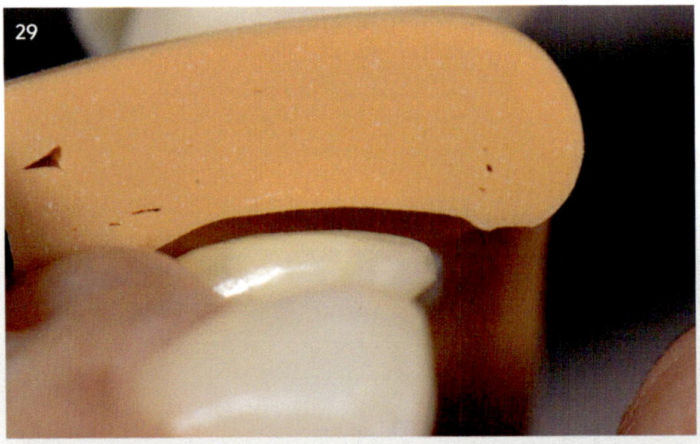
29

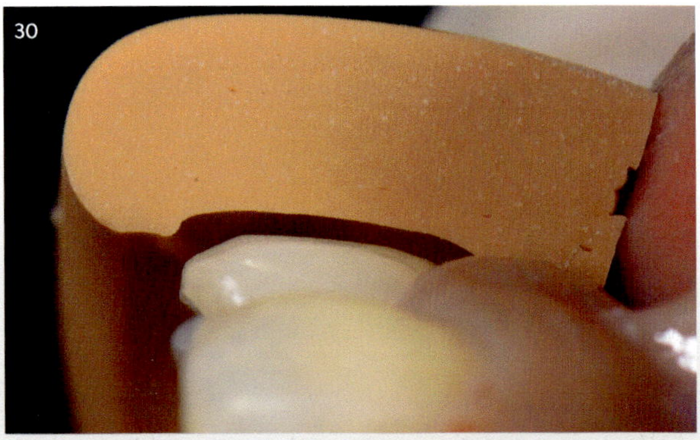
30

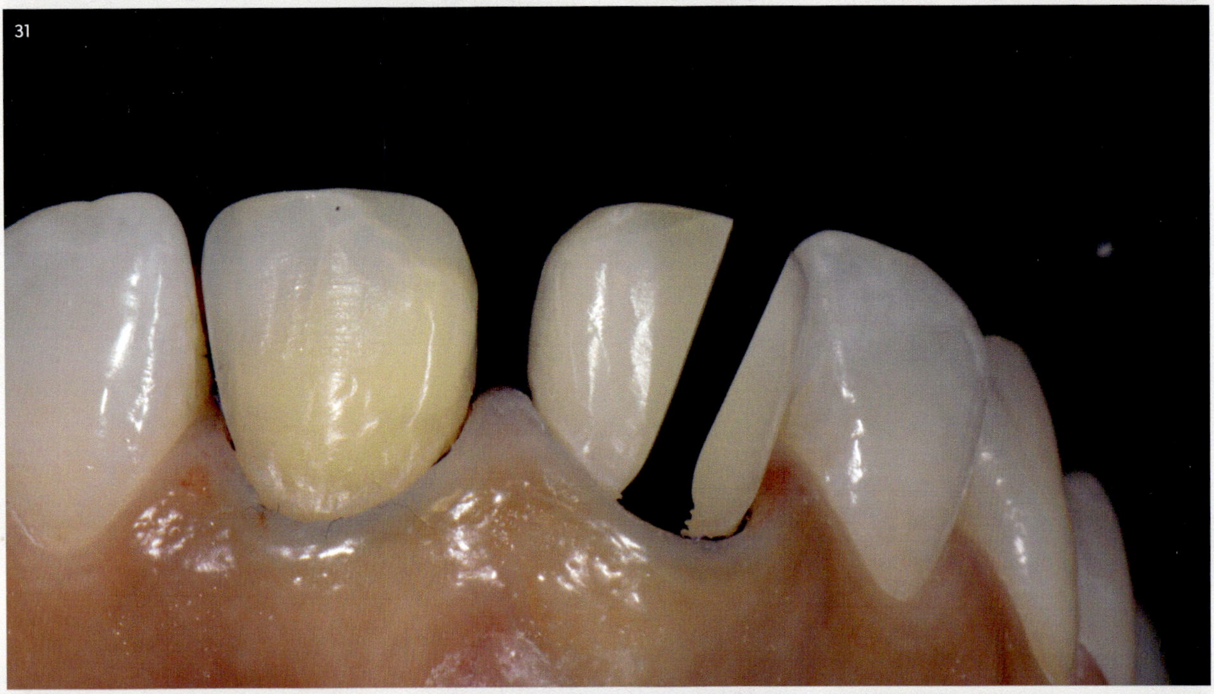
31

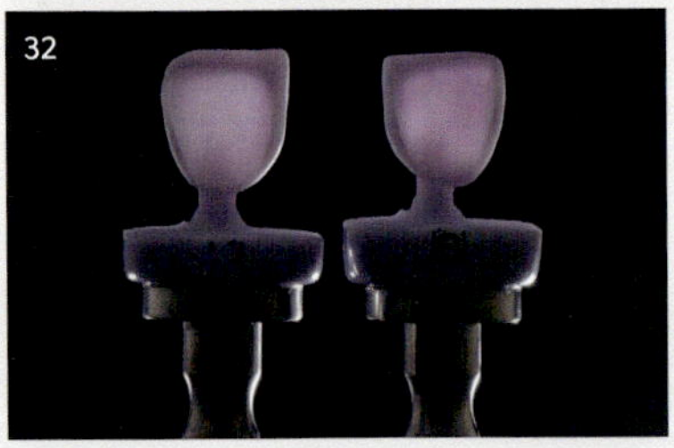
32

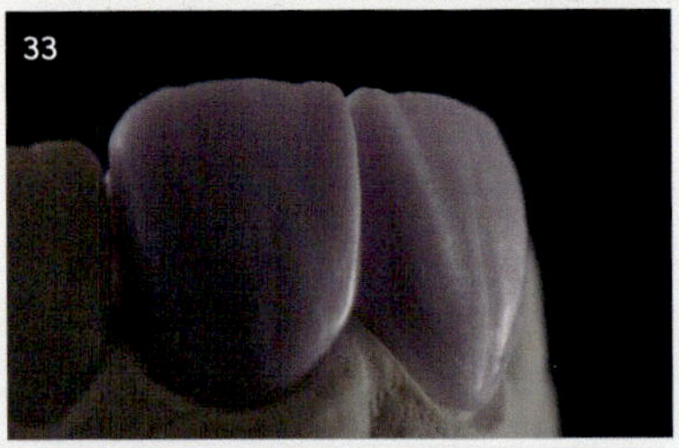
33

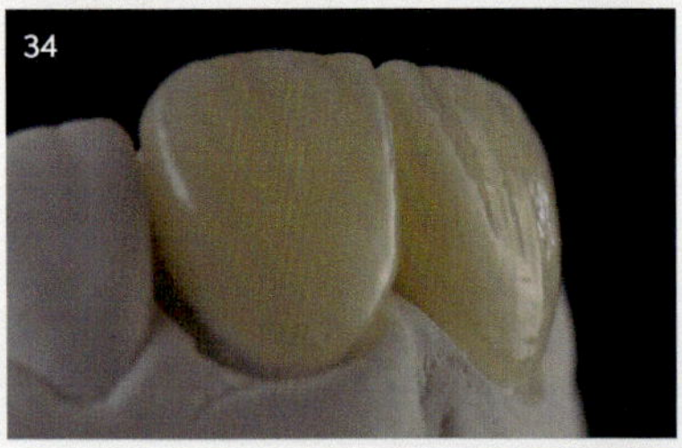
34

Figure 35 Initial situation.

Figure 36 Final situation, note how the color of 11 an 21 match perfectly.

Figure 37 Comparison between the target color (tooth 12) and the final color (tooth 11). Color difference is lower than 1,6 DE, which corresponds to an excellent match.

Figure 38 Comparison between the two centrals, where the color difference corresponds to a perfect match between centrals; the dark substrate is perfectly masked off.

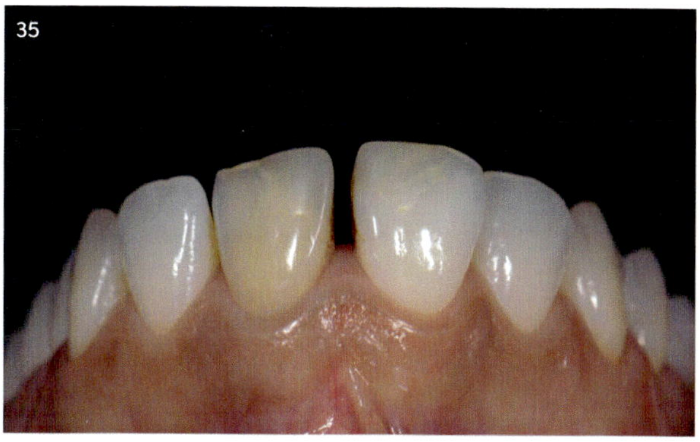
35

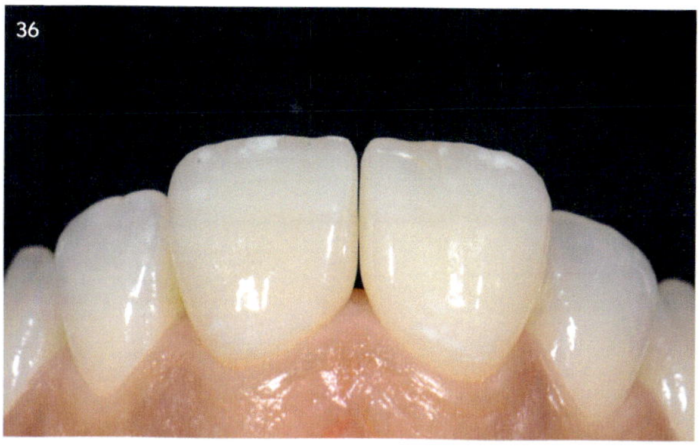
36

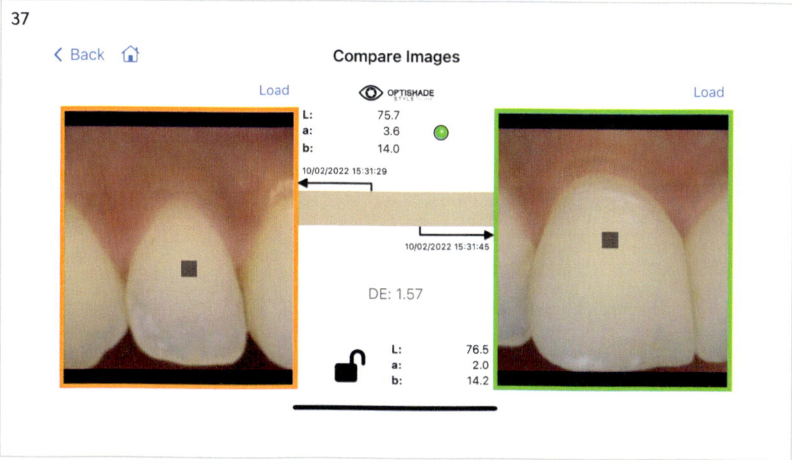

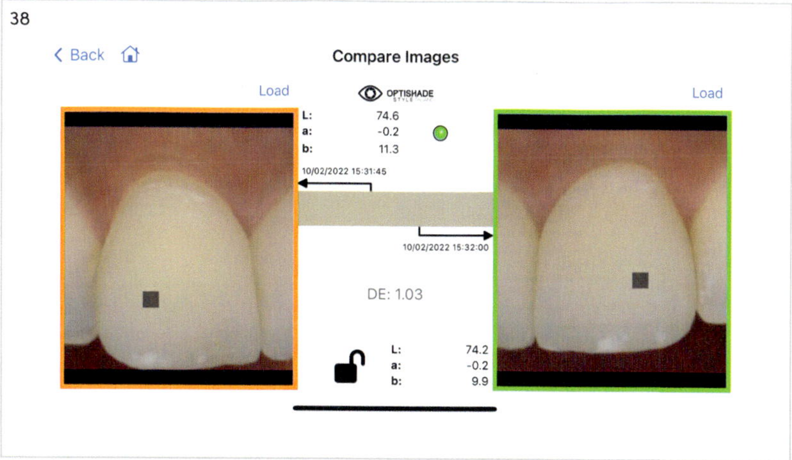

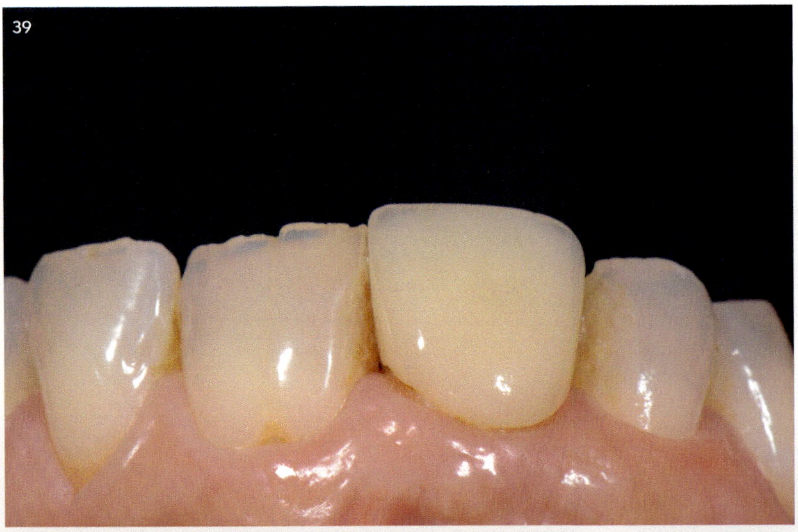

Figure 39 Initial situation: the patient asks for help to solve smile alignment and crown ageing.

Figures 40–41 After project design and mock-up, the clinician proceeds to crown removal and three laminates are prepared.

Figure 42 Once the analogical impression has been received, the plaster model is prepared to highlight all details.

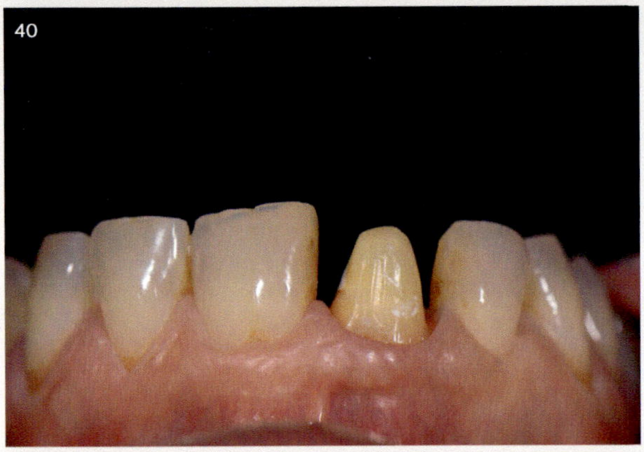

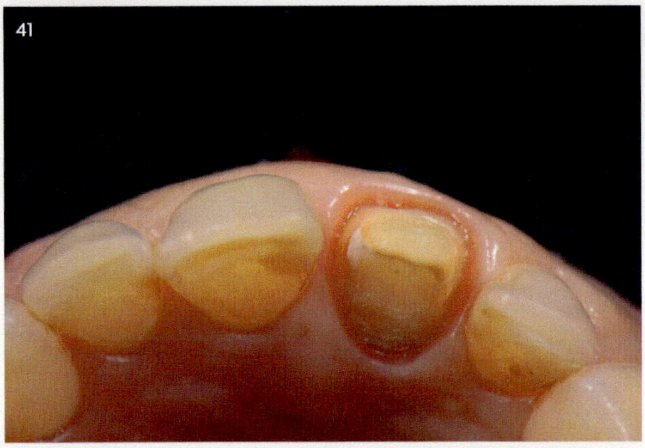

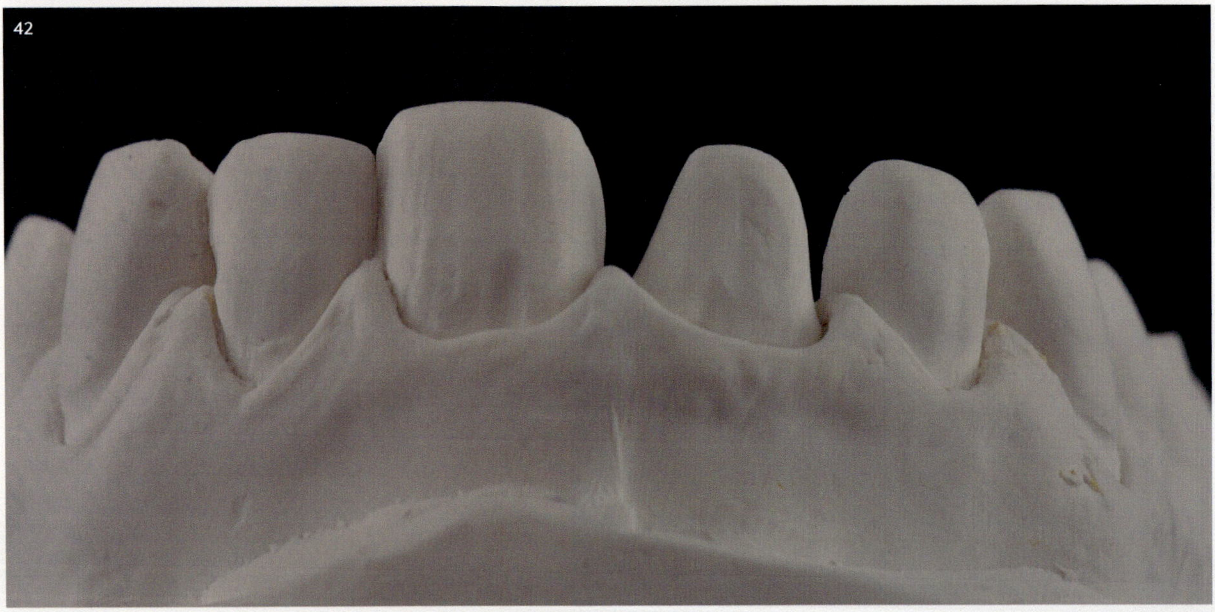

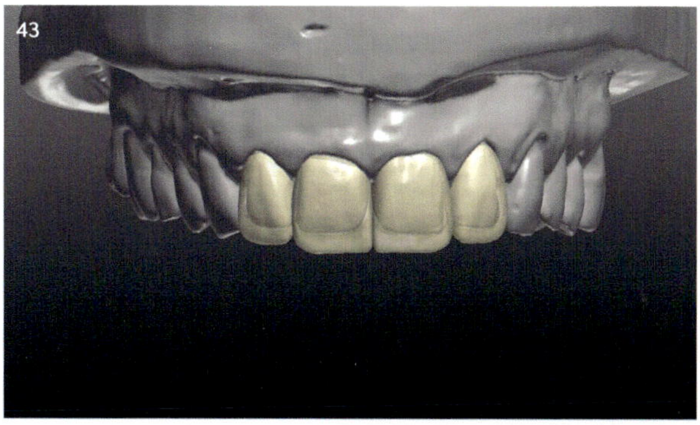

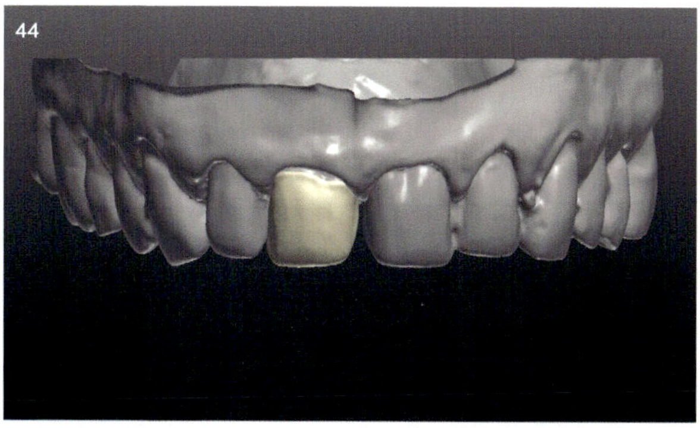

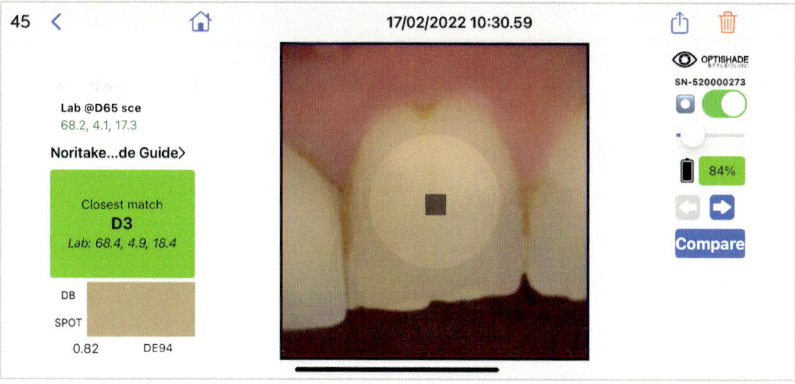

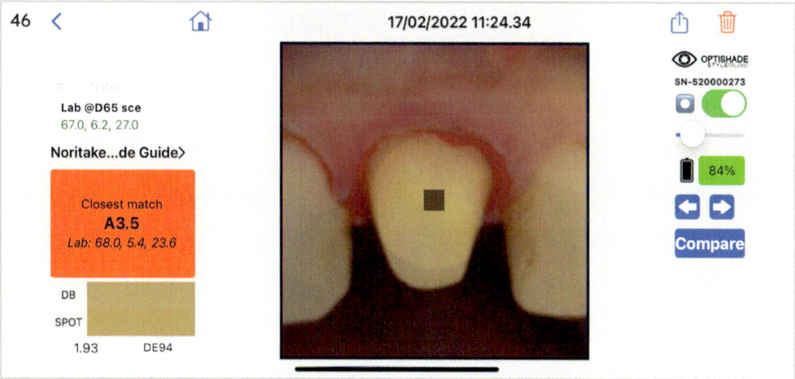

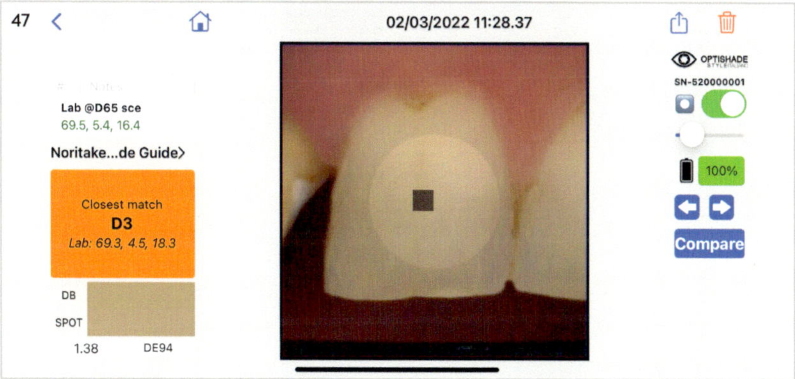

Figures 43–44 After scanning, the initial model is uploaded to the software for matching, and modeling for a cut-back crown, which is prepared by copying the shape of the natural central tooth as prepared beforehand. Thus, a homogenous situation is created.

Figures 45–46–47 In this case, Optishade proves to be helpful to achieve an ideal aesthetic solution[6]. The clinician collects the relevant data from the natural tooth. The abutment color and the prepped tooth color are also assessed so that not only the final requested color[7], but also the sub-layer color from the natural teeth are recorded. All these accurate details[8] will evidently characterize the final result. All the aforesaid evaluations will be useful to determine the color of the zirconia cut-back crown.

Figures 48–49–50–51 Before sending the finalized job back to the clinic, in order to carry out all the necessary color checks in lab, a PMMA aesthetic model will be manufactured. This will allow in-lab optical assessment of the zirconia crown so that, after porcelain correction, it will perfectly match the natural substrate shade. As we can see in the last picture of this series, we are using 3-Paste to help the clinician select and assess the best color shade when cementing.

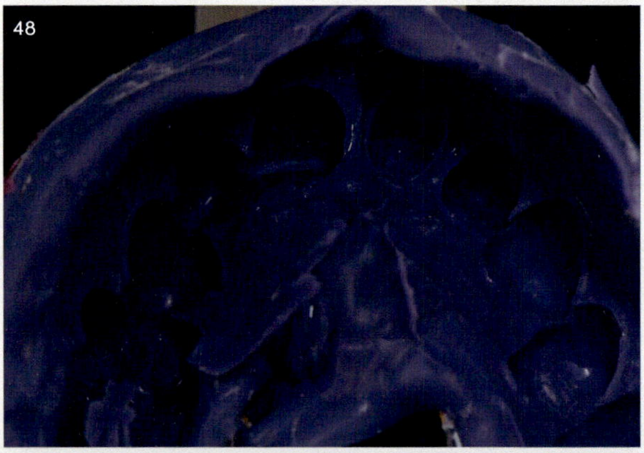

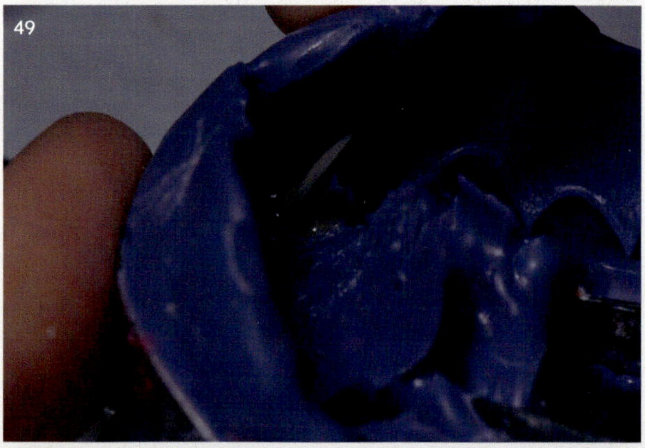

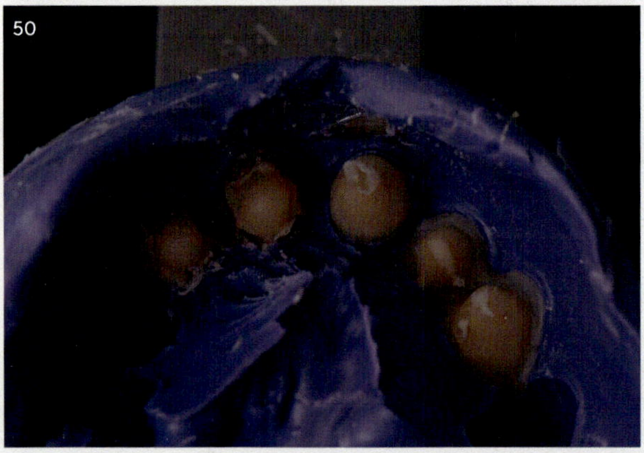

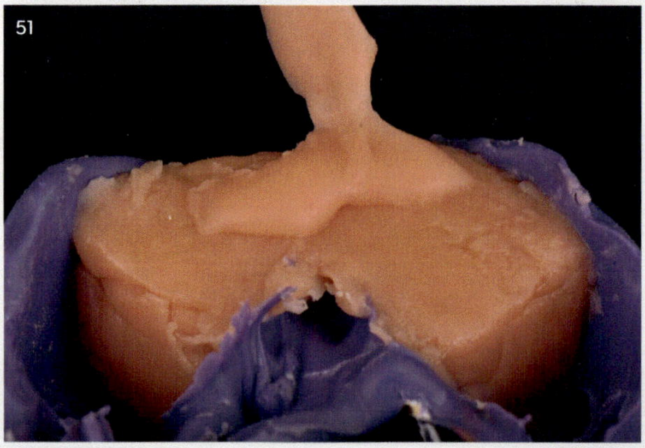

Figures 52–53–54–55–56–57 However, as the clinician took an analogical impression earlier on, we can also rely on the gypsum master model for further precision checks on the final job. In this case, we will proceed to the correction of the substrate of the zirconia crown by means of traditional porcelain. The target of this further step is to correct the zirconia crown so that it will perfectly replicate the adjacent natural abutment. So, both substrates will "optically influence" the porcelain laminates that will be manufactured to complete the project.

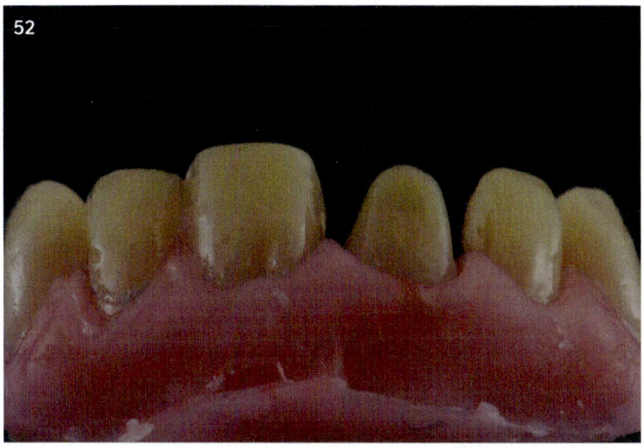
52

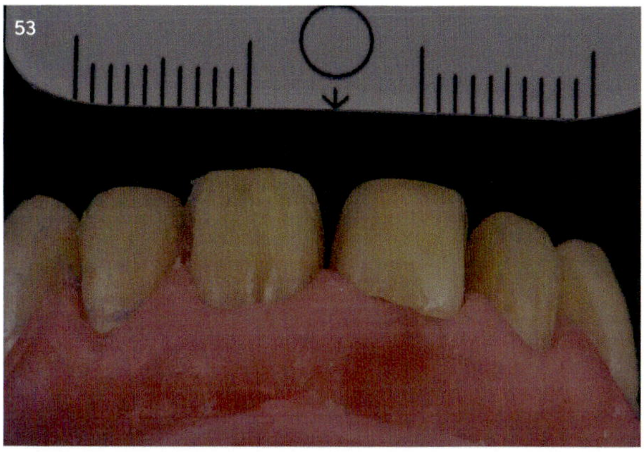
53

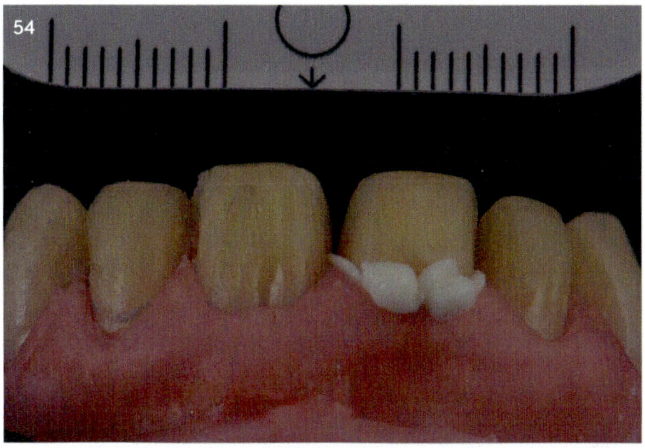
54

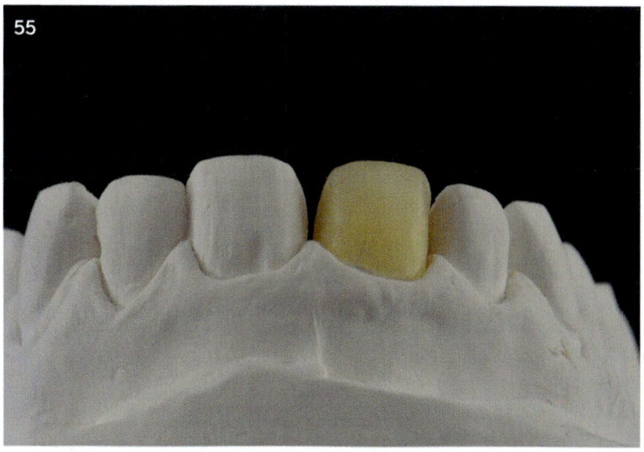
55

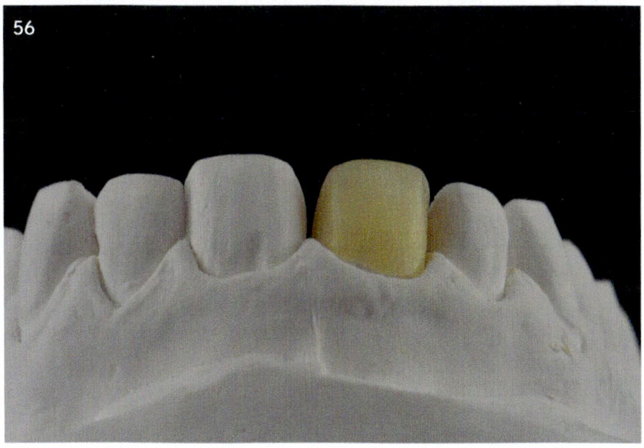
56

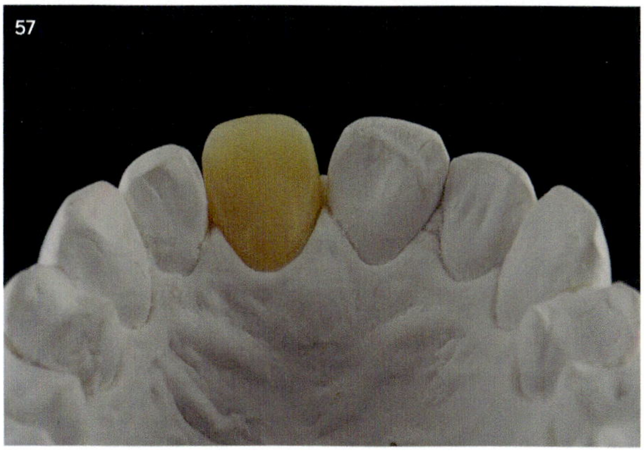
57

58

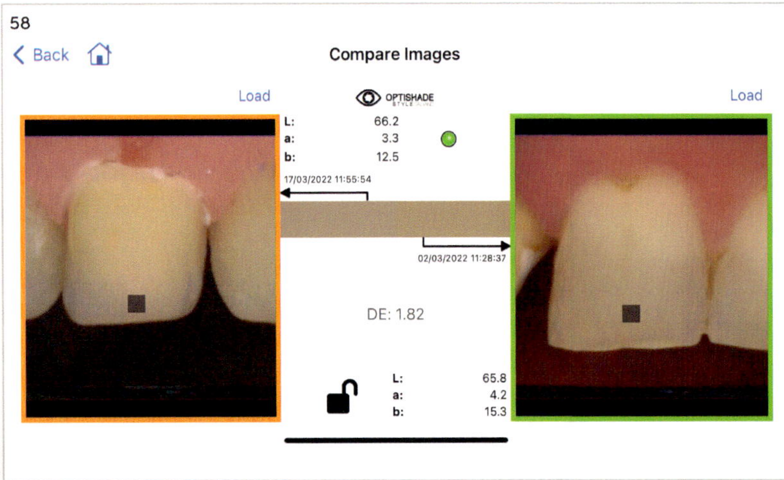

59

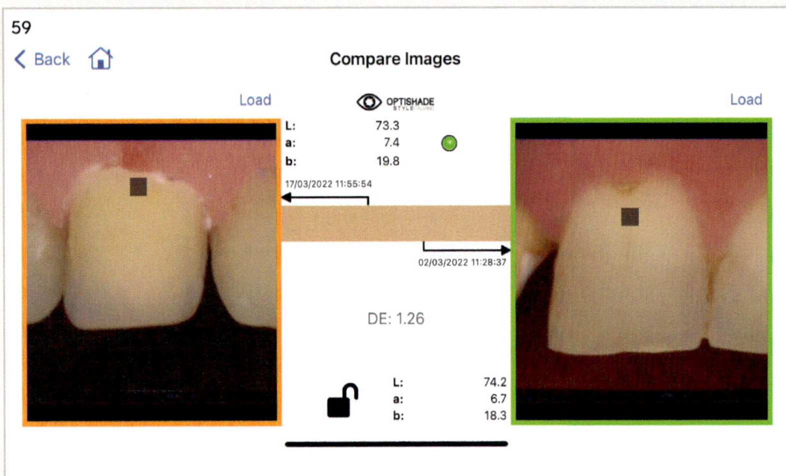

Figures 58–59 After baking the ceramic we will assess the final result by comparison with the natural tooth[9]. The DE will be evaluated and, if acceptable (see table), we can proceed to the next step.

Figure 60 We are now ready to mill the lithium disilicate and, before crystallization, we will proceed to the fitting phase on the master model.

60

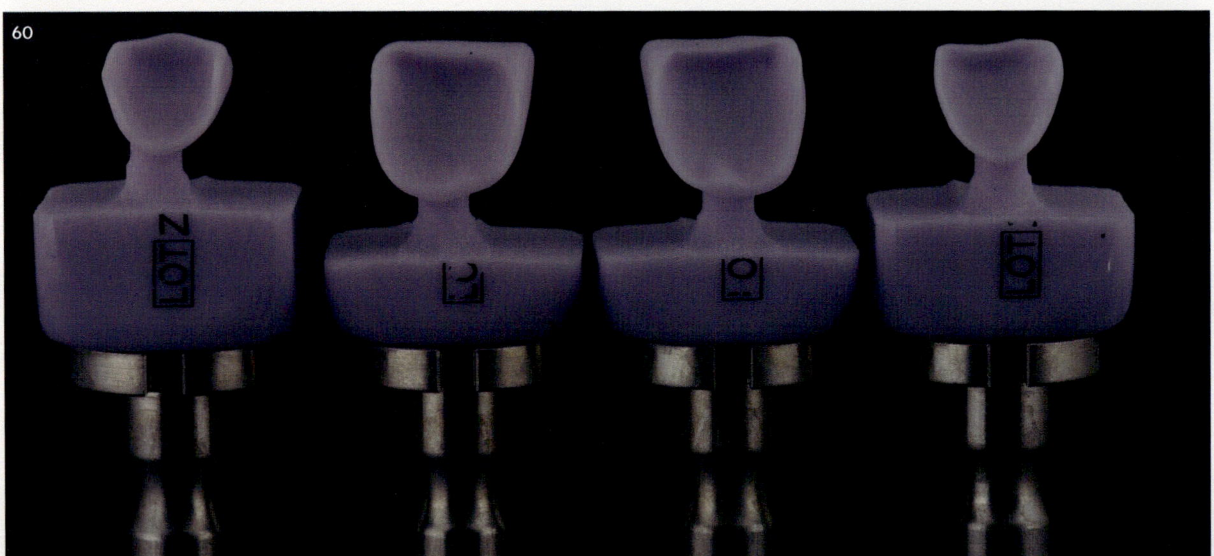

Figures 61–62 This is the result after crystallization[10], as adapted on the master model.

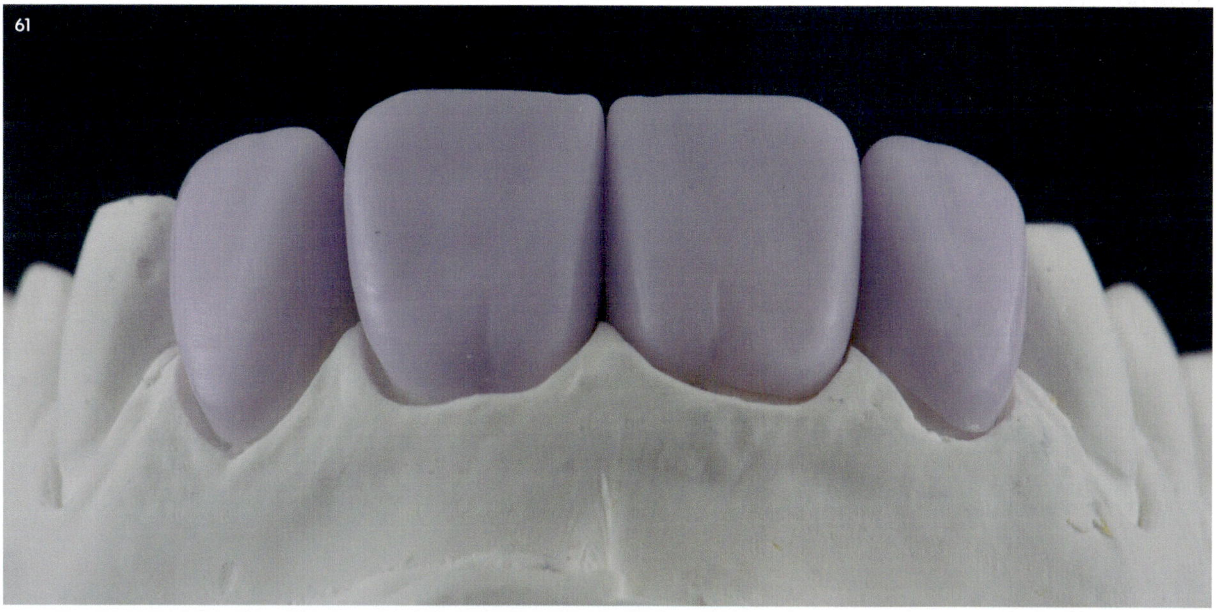

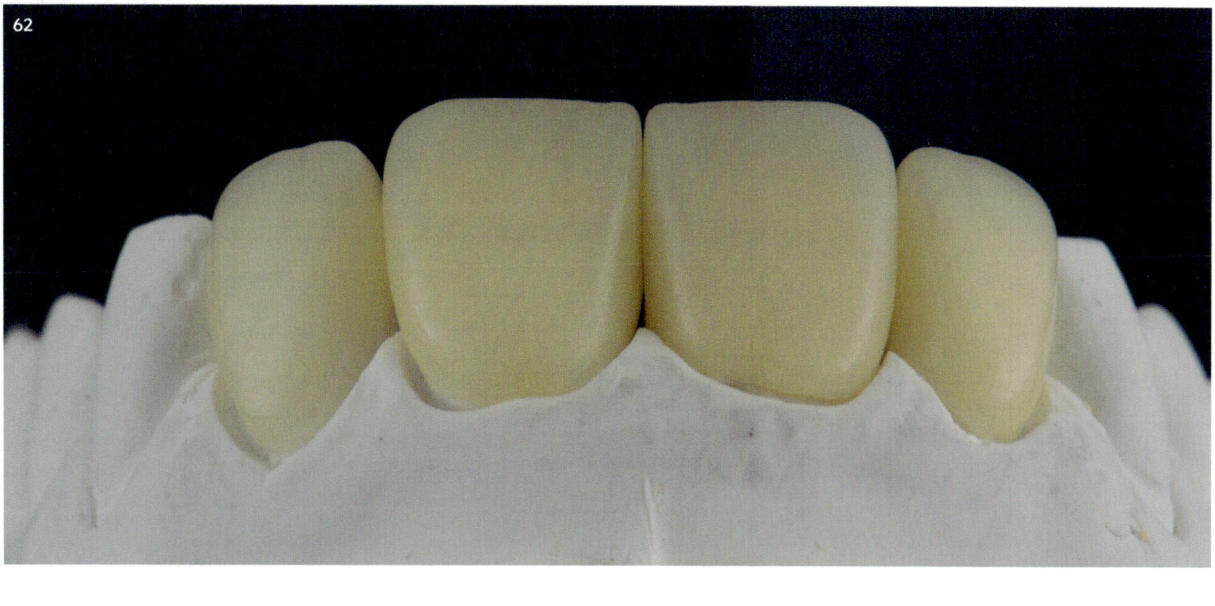

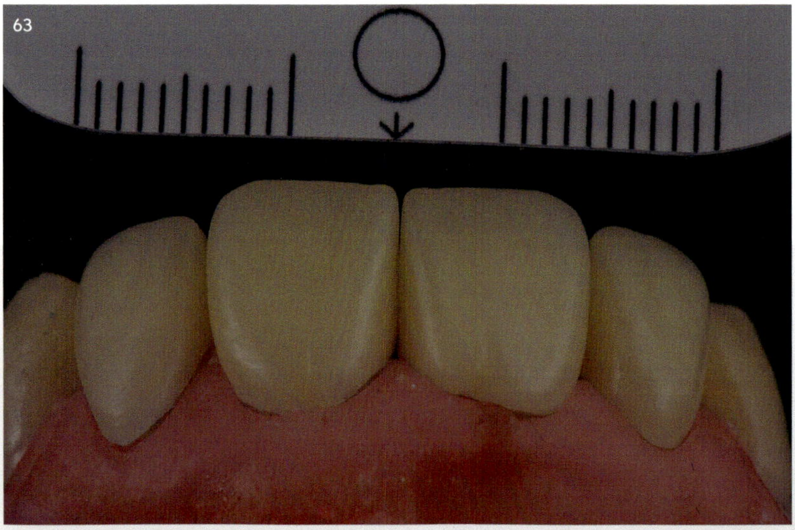

Figures 63–64–65–66–67 For optical evaluation, all the facets will be fitted onto the aesthetic model[11]. Here, corrections on the incisal sides are needed—whereas the DE in the cervical area is fine.

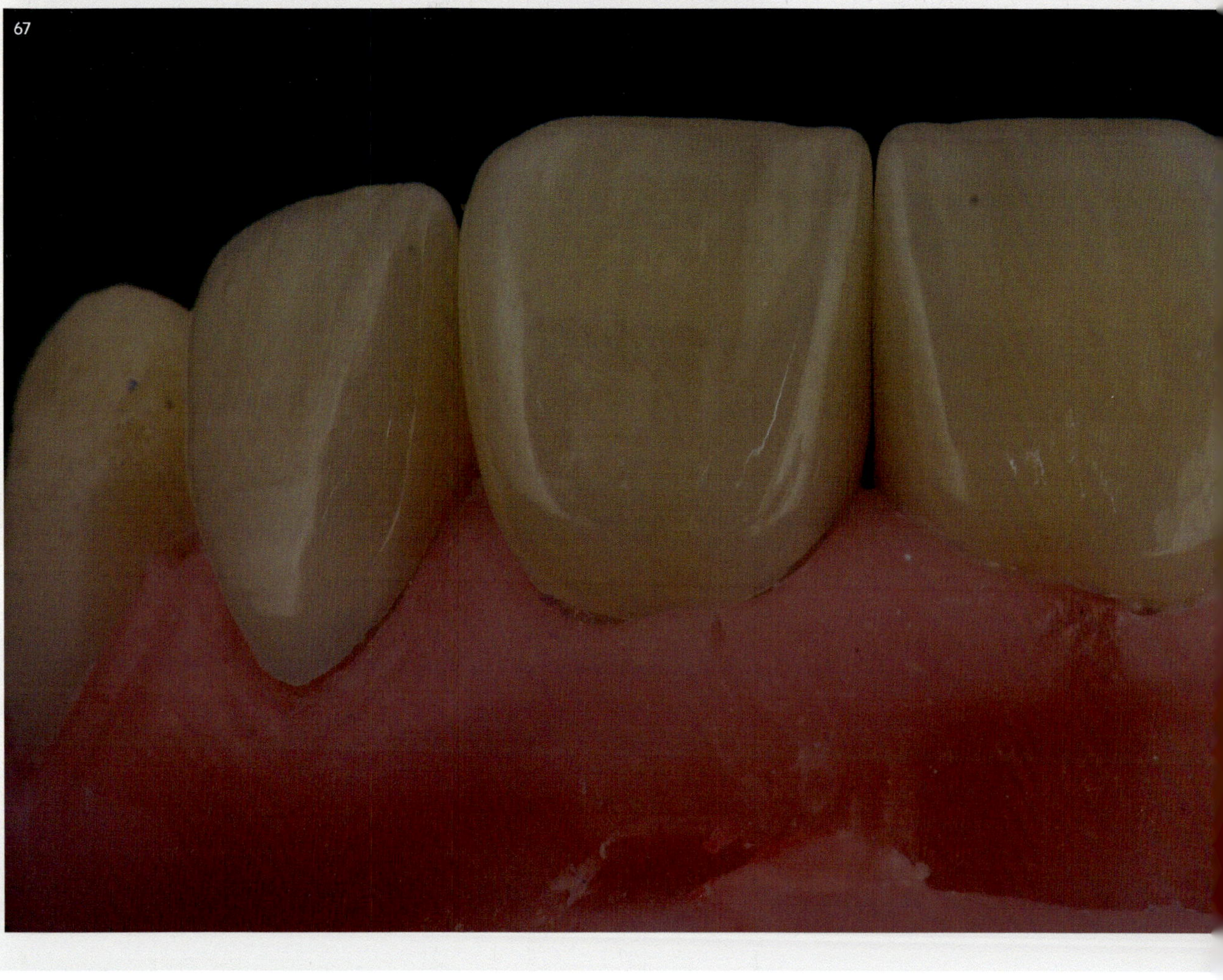

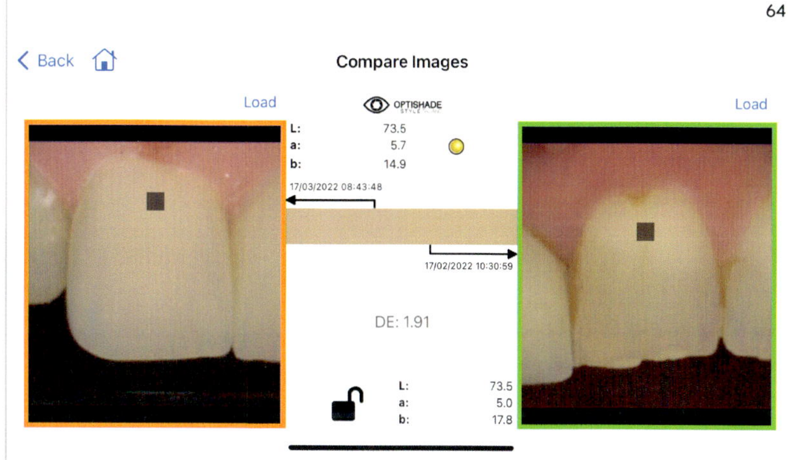
Back
Compare Images
Load
OPTISHADE
Load
L: 73.5
a: 5.7
b: 14.9
17/03/2022 08:43:48
17/02/2022 10:30:59
DE: 1.91
L: 73.5
a: 5.0
b: 17.8

64

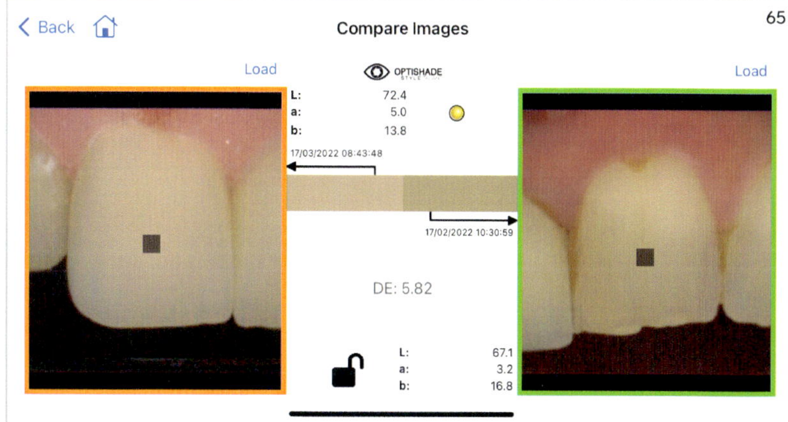
Back
Compare Images
Load
OPTISHADE
Load
L: 72.4
a: 5.0
b: 13.8
17/03/2022 08:43:48
17/02/2022 10:30:59
DE: 5.82
L: 67.1
a: 3.2
b: 16.8

65

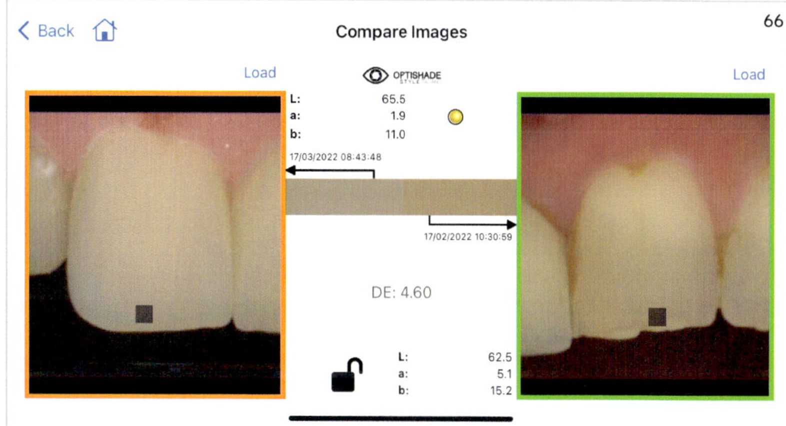
Back
Compare Images
Load
OPTISHADE
Load
L: 65.5
a: 1.9
b: 11.0
17/03/2022 08:43:48
17/02/2022 10:30:59
DE: 4.60
L: 62.5
a: 5.1
b: 15.2

66

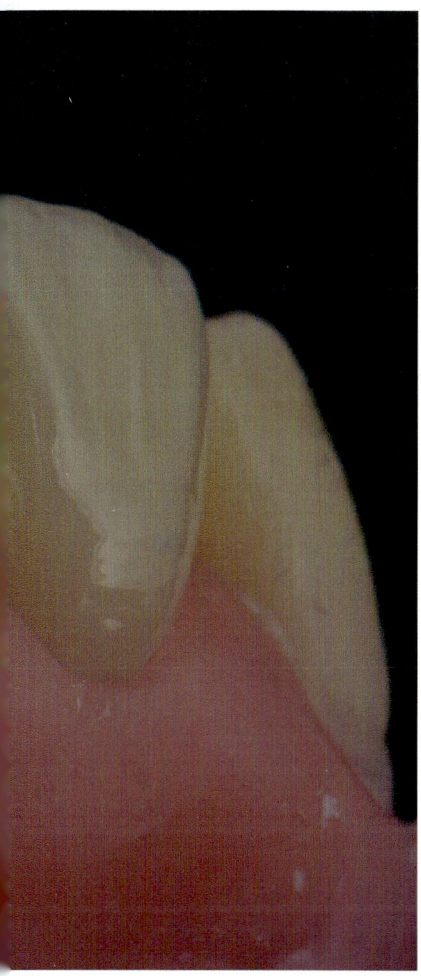

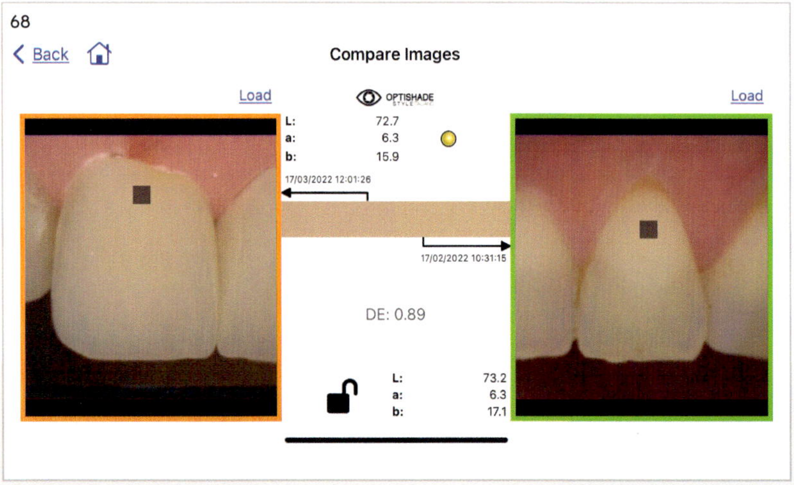

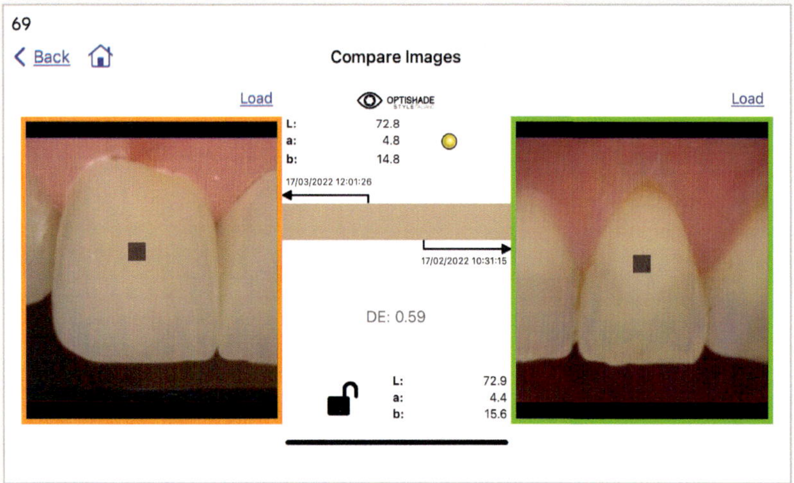

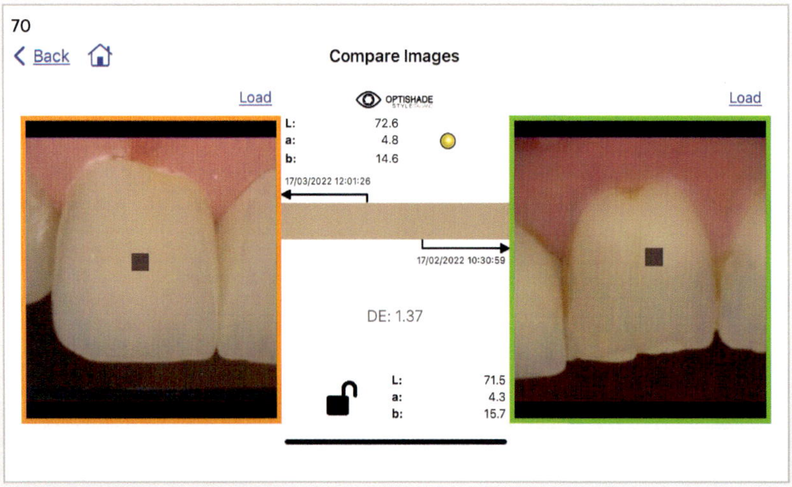

Figures 68–69–70 In-lab quality control. Here is the corrected comparison with an acceptable DE. Through in-lab Optishade quality check, further in-clinic color assessment sessions can be avoided.

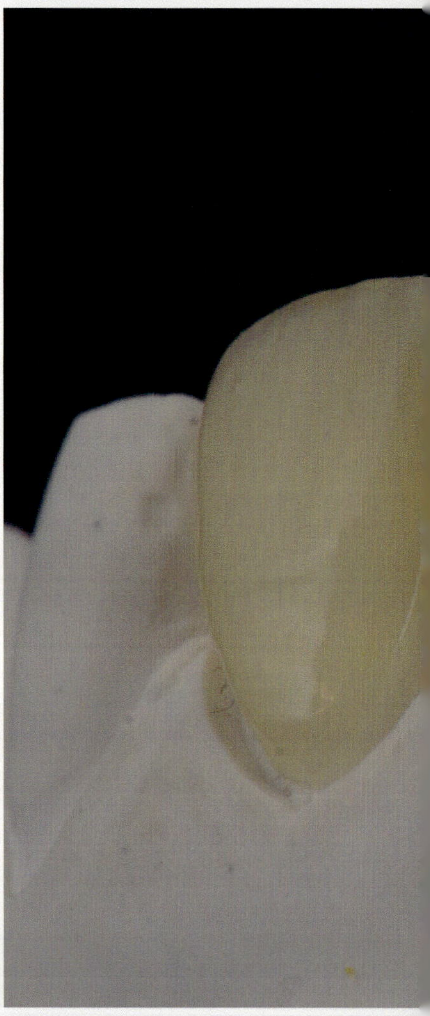

Figure 71 Before final delivery, a further precision check of all the parts will be carried out on the master model.

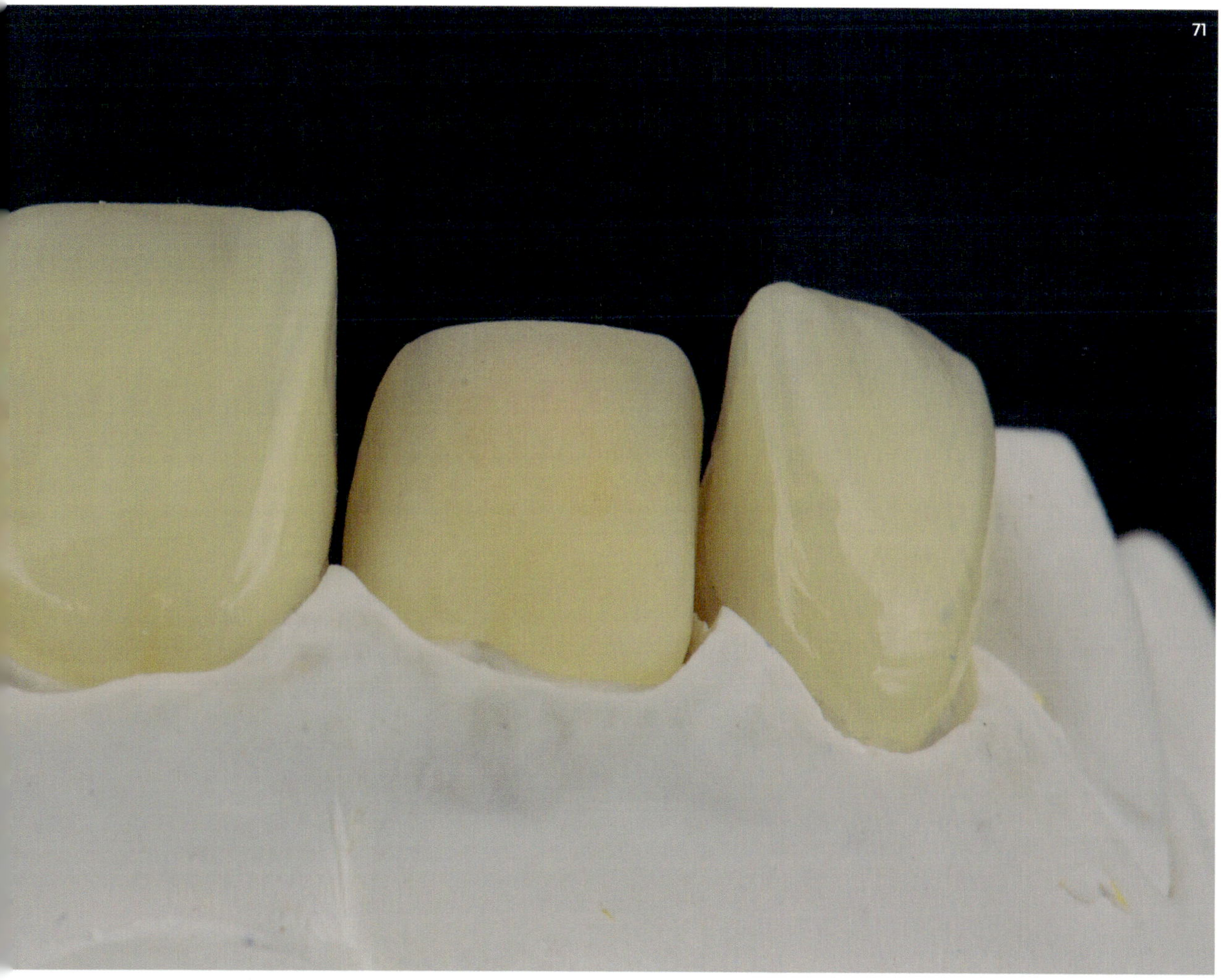

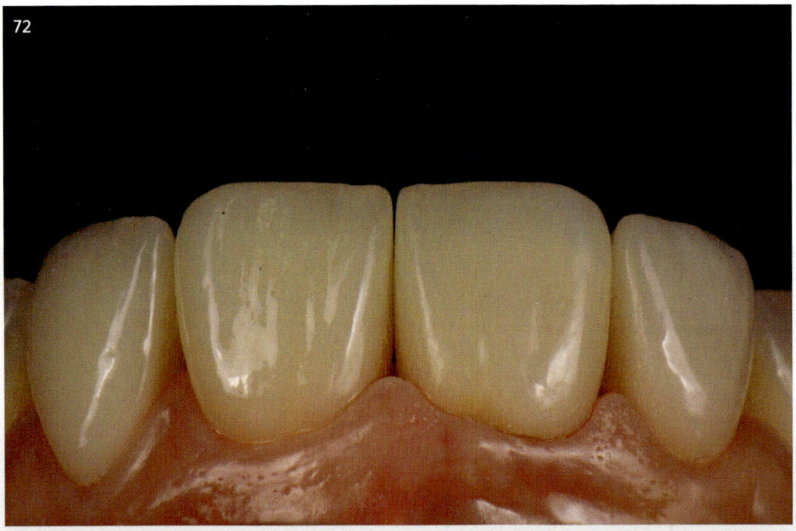

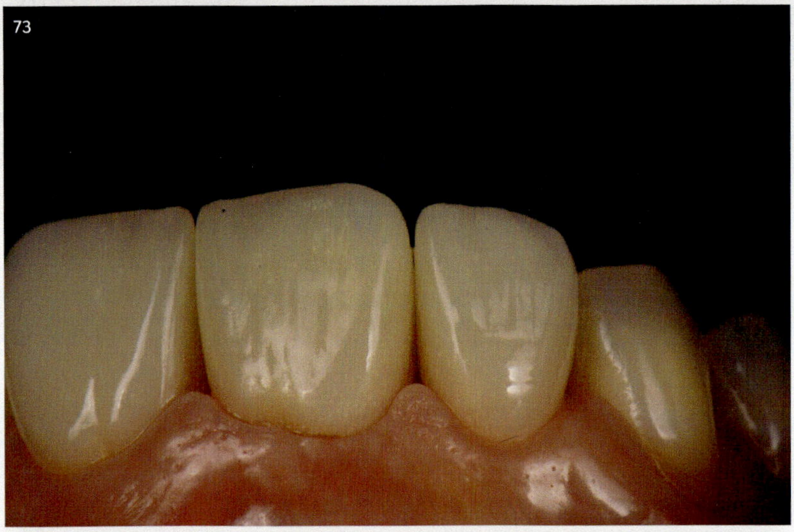

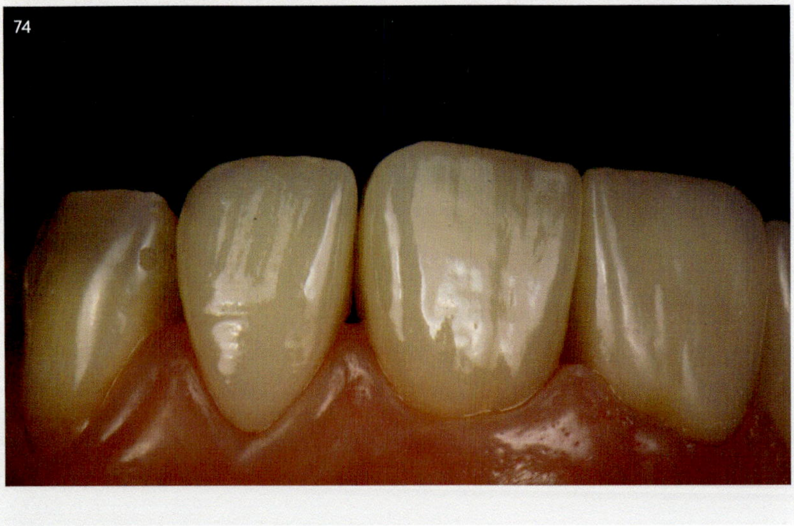

Figures 72–73–74 The finalized job is then fitted into the mouth. The bonding phase will take great advantage of the previous Optishade in-lab precision checks.

CONCLUSIONS

Digital color removes the subjectivity of the eye. As long as the measure is correctly taken, the colorimeter cannot be fooled as the human eye.
Communication through numbers is the most precise way to achieve objective color assessment.
With precise data, we can calculate ceramic mixing, layering, and much more.
Besides being precise and accurate, new technologies are now user-friendly, easy-to-share, and safe, moreover they are universal and guarantee long-term top reliability.

BIBLIOGRAPHY

1. Manauta J, Salat A. Devoto W, Putignano A. *Layers2, The StyleItaliano clinical secrets.* Quintessence pub. 2022.
2. Browning WD, Contreras-Bulnes R, Brackett MG, Brackett WW. Color differences: polymerized composite and corresponding Vitapan Classical shade tab. *J Dent.* 2009;37.34-9.
3. Paravina RD, Westland S, Imai FH, Kimura M, Powers JM. Evaluation of blending effect of composites related to restoration size. *Dent Mater.* 2006;(4):299-307. Miller L. Organizing color in dentistry. *J Am Dent Assoc.* 1987; (spec issue):26E-40E.
4. Paravina RD, Pereira Sanchez NA, Tango RN, Harmonization of color measurements for dental application. *Color Research and application Journal.* 2020;45(Issue 6):1094-1100.
5. Rizzi A, Bonanomi C, Brazzoli S, Cerutti A & Kovacs-Vajna ZM. Assessing appearance in human dental colour space, *Computer Methods in Biomechanics and Biomedical Engineering: Imaging & Visualization.* 2016:1, 59-67.
6. Douglas RD, Steinhauer TJ, Wee AG Intraoral Determination of the tolerance of dentists for perceptibility and acceptability of shade mismatch. *Journal of Prosthetic Dentistry.* 2007;97:200-8.
7. Paravina RD, Pérez MM, Ghinea R. Acceptability and perceptibility thresholds in dentistry: A comprehensive review of clinical and research applications. *J Esthet Restor Dent.* 2019;31(2):103-112.
8. Wee AG, Lindsey DT, Shroyer KM, Johnston WM. Use of a porcelain color discrimination test to evaluate color difference formulas. *Journal of Prosthetic Dentistry.* 2007;98:101-9.
9. Paravina RD, Ghinea R, Herrera LJ, Bona AD, Igiel C, Linninger M, Sakai M, Takahashi H, Tashkandi E, Perez Mdel M. Color difference thresholds in dentistry. *J Esthet Restor Dent.* 2015;27 Suppl 1:S1-9.
10. Malacara D. *Color Vision and colorimetry*, Second edition. Spie Press. 2011. 16-8, 75-6, 91-97.
11. Berns R. *Billmeyer and Saltzman's Principles of Color Technology*, fourth edition. Wiley. 2019. 42-5, 51, 74-5, 92-105, 111-144, 212-14.

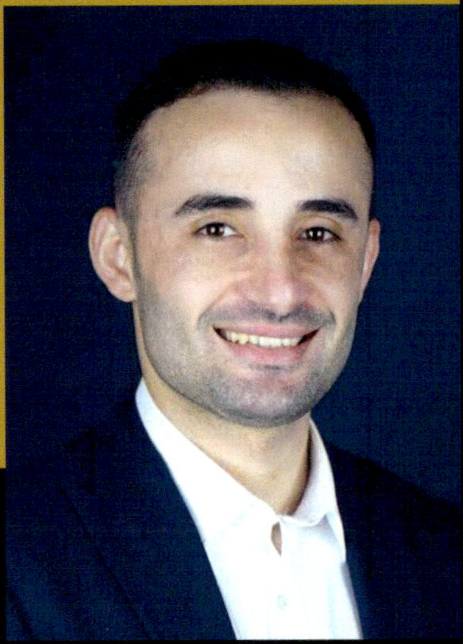

OSAMA SHAALAN

Palestine

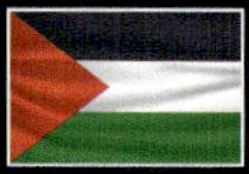

Born in Palestine the 12/03/1988; graduated with an excellent honors degree in Dental Medicine in 2013 at Sinai University, since he graduated his interest has been in restorative and aesthetic dentistry because he believes in the idea that everyone deserves to have a beautiful and healthy smile Irrespective of their economic backgrounds.

Dr Shaalan maintained his clinical practice in aesthetics and restorative dentistry in his private clinic in Palestine. He is an international lecturer for aesthetic and restorative dentistry and gives many lectures locally and internationally focused on his passion for direct composite restorations and how to use simplified techniques and materials in daily work to make smile makeovers fast, repeatable, and predictable.

He is also a course director in Palestine, as he gave many courses for local dentists and international dentists about direct composite techniques and other topics in the field of aesthetics dentistry.

Participation as a speaker and representing his country in many international conferences in Bulgaria, Spain, Germany, Italy, Turkey, Dubai, Egypt, Libya, and Austria.

He is awarded by StyleItaliano in 2018 as the best follower award in the community sharing the same philosophy and passion of StyleItaliano in Madrid (Spain) at 300k the congress.

He is awarded as the first gold Member of StyleItaliano in Sofia (Bulgaria) at StyleItaliano meeting in parallel with the Sofia Dental meeting, because of his participation and contributions to the community and sharing StyleItaliano philosophy towards patients and dentists.

He is selected to be a country chairperson for Palestine at the European society of cosmetic dentistry in Rome (Italy).

Author of many articles and a publisher in the field of aesthetics dentistry at StyleItaliano FMC-London and Dentistry- UK magazine.

Co-author of one chapter of *Layers 2* book, *Direct Composites: The StyleItaliano Clinical Secrets.*

Part of the StyleItaliano developing team and key opinion leader of many international dental companies.

The inventor of a posterior replica instrument for direct posterior composite modeling and occlusal shaping of posterior teeth.

SMILE MAKEOVER WITH DIRECT COMPOSITE VENEERS

When talking about anterior teeth, the conversation often will be about aesthetics, as it's needed in daily life for self-confidence, social integration, everyday relationships, and job opportunities[1]. The problem is when the patients come in with an unpleasant smile due to many clinical situations such as a problem in the color or the shape of the teeth which causes an impairment of the smile harmony[2,3]. The use of direct composite restorations is considered a reliable treatment as in the last years there has been a massive evolution in composite resins, adhesive systems, and restorative techniques that has led to a significant improvement in daily clinical work[4,5,22]. The adhesive properties of the composite resin, the minimal preparation, and the aesthetic appearance are the three main advantages of composite resin in the anterior area[6,7,11]. However, there are challenges during working with cases of multiple direct anterior restorations in daily work, the time of the procedure, the amount of stress[8,9], and dentists' skills[10]. All these factors make the practitioners think carefully before choosing direct restoration as a treatment option.
This chapter will describe the StyleItaliano philosophy for Simplified direct veneering in a predictable and repeatable way and how to overcome daily work challenges.

STYLEITALIANO PHILOSOPHY for multiple direct anterior restorations (the simplified approach)

1. WDB CompoSite system (Optident, UK).
2. SOLO anterior (LM-arte, Finland).
3. Unica matrix (Polydentia, Switzerland).
4. Lucida polishing (Diashine, USA).

StyleItaliano has introduced new simple smart tools and materials for making direct restorations very simple and fast, even in complex cases.

This approach aims to

- Minimizing the procedure time. Instead of doing multiple direct cases from 3–4 hours, using this instruments, the practitioner can do the same work in 1–2 hours.
- Making the cases in a single visit without a wax-up step, thus decreasing the time and the fees.

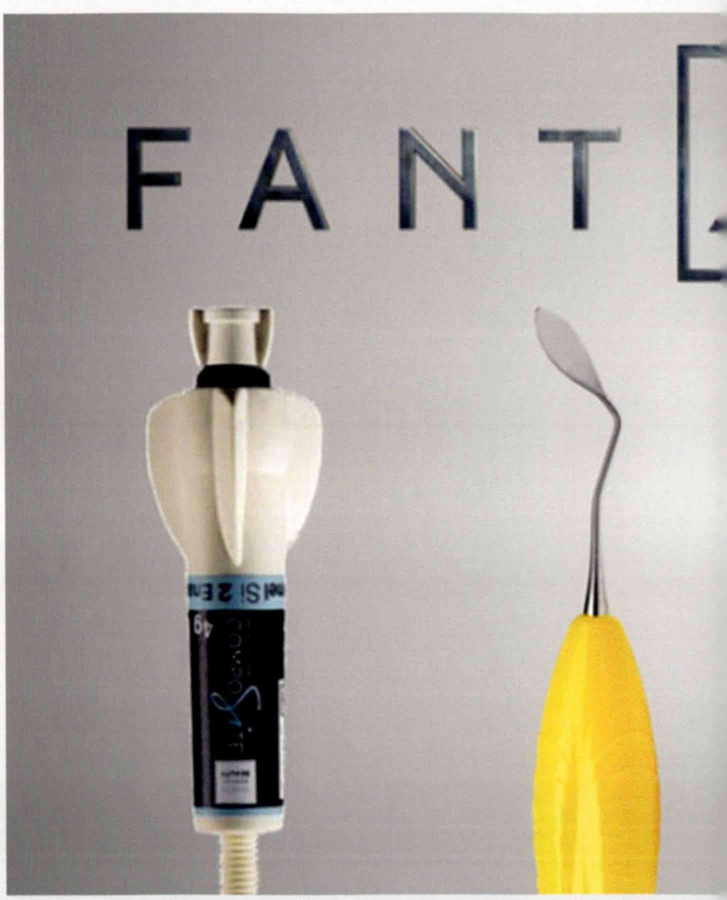

- Predicting the results very easily in a repeatable way.
- Minimizing the number of instruments and materials that are used.
- Minimizing the steps to complete the entire procedure and require minimal levels of skills.
- Decreasing the stress during work and increase the quality of the final result.

How can the dentist achieve this?

This can be done using essential materials and tools especially designed by StyleItaliano for direct veneering cases or any direct anterior composite restorations by (1):

1. Restoring with a simple composite system using WDB CompoSite system (Optident, UK).
2. Using one matrix for all anterior restorations with Unica matrix (Polydentia, Switzerland).
3. Handling and manipulating with one instrument for all anterior restorations with Solo anterior (LM-arte, Finland).
4. Using simplified finishing and one final step of polishing-Lucida polishing (Diashine, USA).

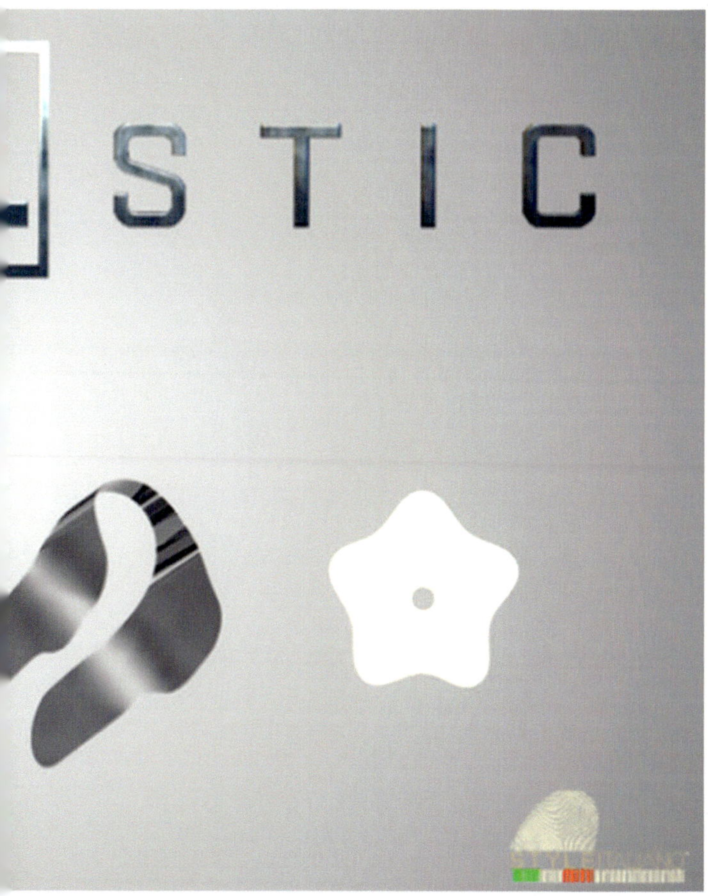

Figure 1 Fantastic 4.

THE FULL APPROACH

This is a case of a young lady who came to the clinic complaining of brown and yellow discolorations, and she needed to have a beautiful and confident smile (2).

There is a mild to moderate fluorosis on her teeth characterized by yellowish-brown discoloration. The treatment of fluorosis depends on the severity of the affected enamel[16]. A retracted view shows that the yellowish-brown discolorations are mainly related to the upper teeth from right canine to left canine. The appearance of teeth affected by mild to moderate fluorosis can be significantly improved by various techniques like bleaching, resin infiltrations, micro-abrasion, direct veneering, or indirect restorations[16,17]. As the patient had limited time and budget, direct veneering suited the patient's needs (3).

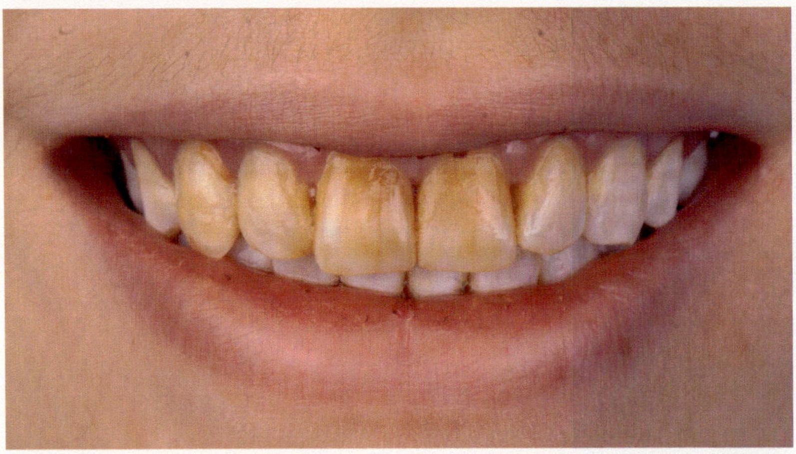

Figure 2 Photo of the initial smile.

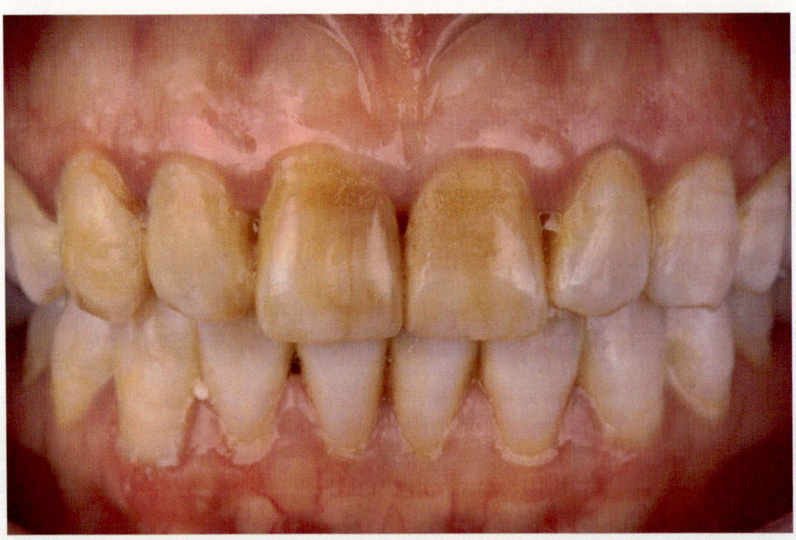

Figure 3 Initial retracted view.

The treatment plan goal is to mask the discolorations and to do a shape correction, especially the incisal embrasures, in an attempt to follow the smile curve to give the illusion of a natural-looking smile[13] (4).

Shade selection using custom shades fabricated from the WDB (UK) CompoSite system, five dentin shades, and only one enamel shade. Select a suitable shade (SI2 Dentin) according to the patient's desire and to complement the harmony of the lower teeth[19] (5).

A little preparation here is mandatory to remove the affected enamel and to enhance the resin-enamel bond strength, because the bonding effectiveness to unground enamel was lower in fluorosis teeth than in prepared teeth[18,23]. This will ensure the application of universal adhesive on sound enamel to improve the resin-enamel bond strength in fluorosis teeth[18] (6).

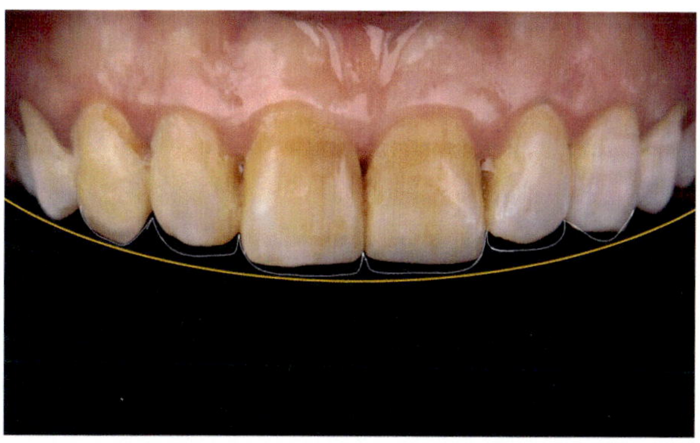

Figure 4 Black contrast view.

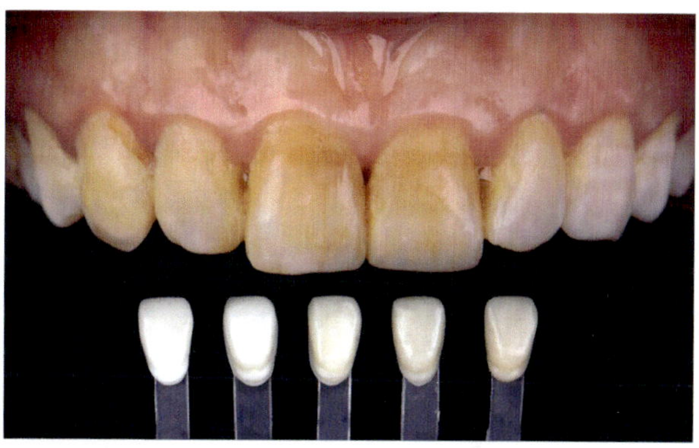

Figure 5 Shade selection photo using custom shade.

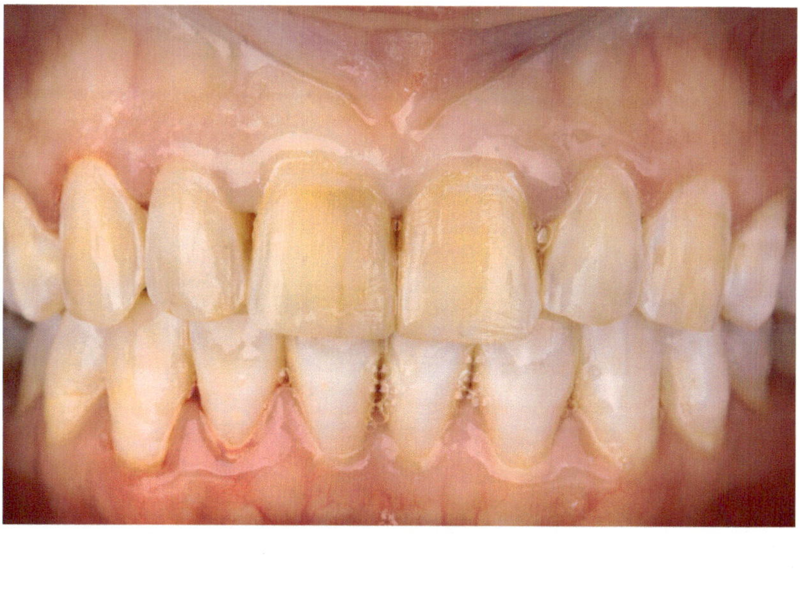

Figure 6 Photo after minimal preparation.

Rubber dam isolation is required to have a clean environment and provide a clear vision. Moreover, it prevents intraoral humidity from affecting adhesion as the bonding performance of adhesive systems depends on the humidity settings[12,25]. The reason for making a split dam technique is because will use Unica matrix to retract and seal the cervical part (7).
Acid etching for 30 seconds by using Scotchbond Universal Etchant (3M ESPE, USA) and washing for 30 seconds to ensure the complete removal of etching gel[12] (8).
The frosty white appearance is a good indicator of enough etching (9).

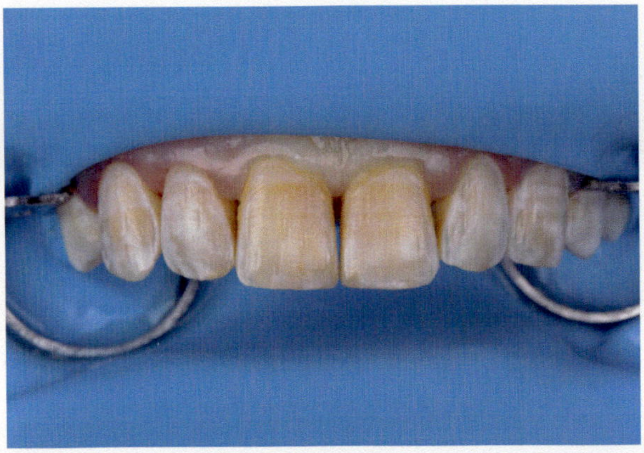

Figure 7 Split dam isolation photo.

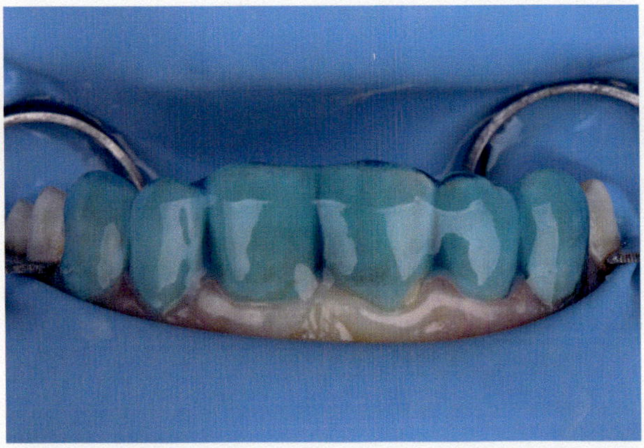

Figure 8 Acid etching.

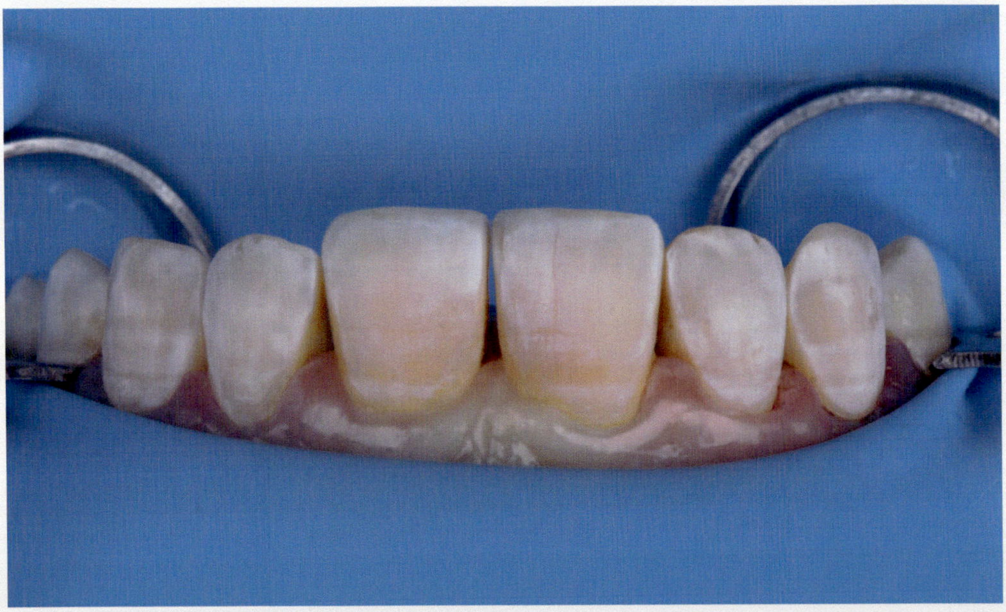

Figure 9 Frosty white after etching.

Universal adhesive application using the Scotchbond Universal bond (3M ESPE, USA) and active rubbing using a brush for 20 seconds against the surface to ensure a complete wetting of the adhesive and the etched enamel (10).
Light curing for 20 seconds using the third-generation CuringPen (Eighteeth, China) (11).
Freehand palatal shell fabrications using the enamel shade (WDB, UK) with a mylar strip supported palatally by a finger (12).

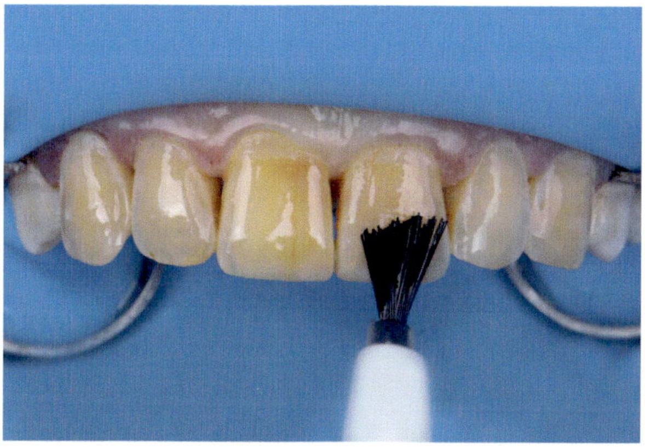

Figure 10 Universal bond application with brush.

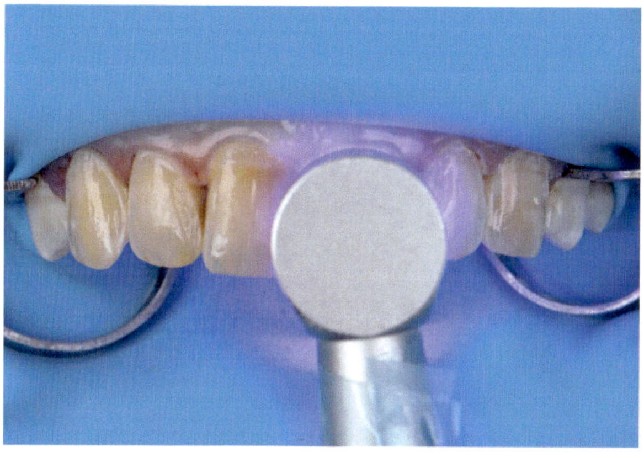

Figure 11 Light curing.

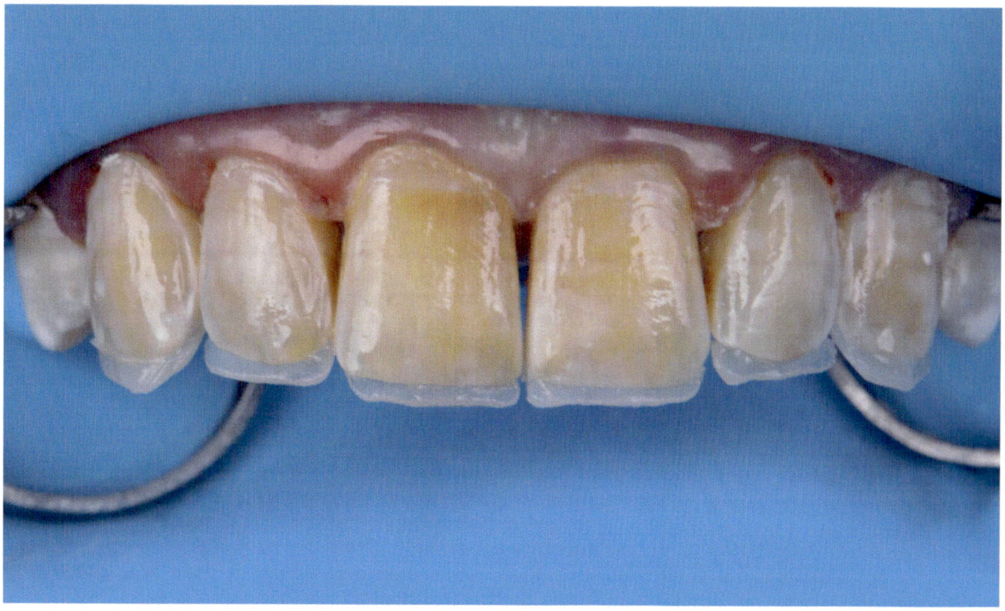

Figure 12 Palatal shell photo.

For multiple anterior restorations, multiple Unica matrix mixtures (Polydentia, Switzerland) can be prepared at the same time. With regular Unica for centrals and minideep for laterals.
One of the advantages of using Unica is the shape can be easily predicted. Furthermore, the symmetry and the midline can be obtained (13).
A Unica frame is produced by building the proximal walls with cervical walls to form the outer contour that will help to predict the final shape of the restorations. In addition to that it will control the amount of composite material during layering, and subsequently decrease the time of the finishing and polishing. Now it's ready to receive the veneering material (14).
During layering composite veneers it is necessary to apply the composite material in one large bulk layer by applying a homogeneous regular mass using the Solo anterior

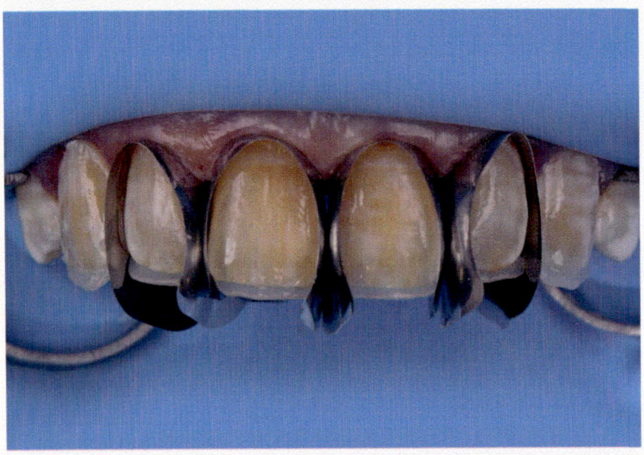

Figure 13 Unica matrix (Polydentia, Switzerland) regular in centrals and minideep in laterals.

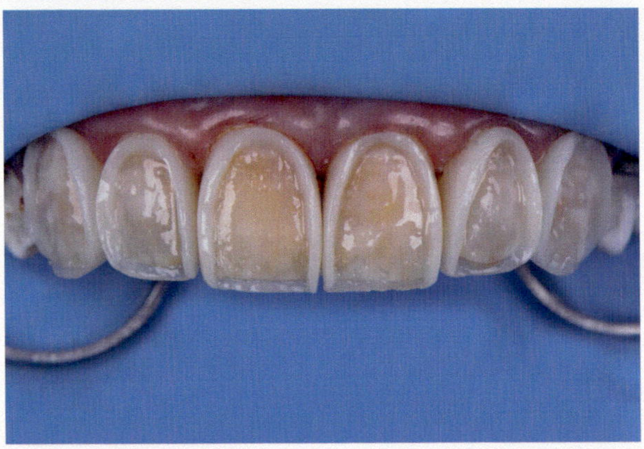

Figure 14 Photo of unica frame.

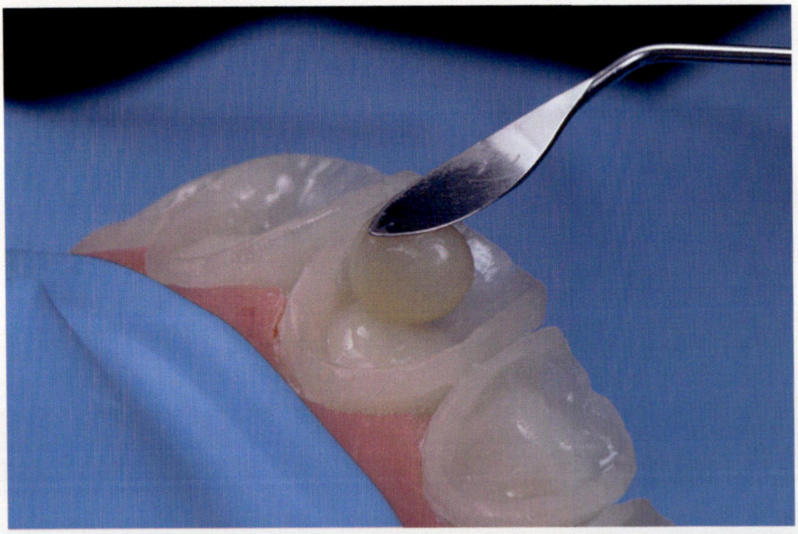

Figure 15 Modeling the veneering layer in a model.

instrument (LM-arte, Finland) on the labial surface. If material is applied incrementally, the possibility of creating voids will be significant, contamination may happen, and multiple layers will need much adaptation for blending the layer[20] (📷 15).

The sharp tip of the straight end is used for mamelons modeling and shaping (📷 16).

The best layering technique in terms of speed and aesthetic results involves using the dentin shade for the entire composite veneers and only the incisal 1\3, which will be characterized with the enamel shade, which means that enamel will cover up to the incisal 1\3. This is fast, simple, and provides a more natural look; better than using two shades dentin and enamel shade for the entire labial surface. In addition, using this recipe will get rid of the enamel thickness issues if increased beyond 0.5 mm[20,21] (📷 17).

After layering the veneering material with the final enamel layer, it is mandatory to have a final smooth surface to enhance the finishing and polishing (📷 18).

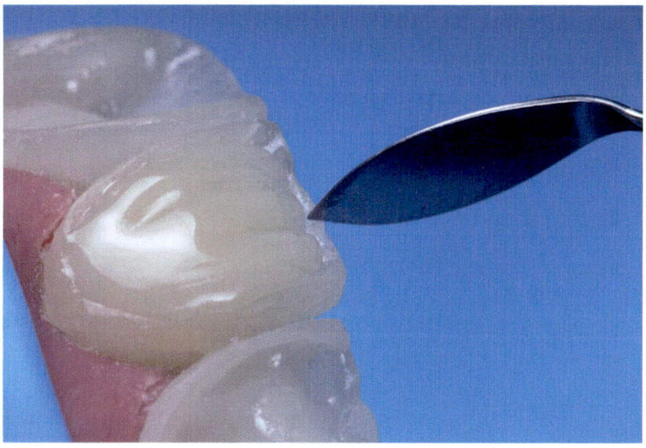

Figure 16 Modeling and shaping mamelons.

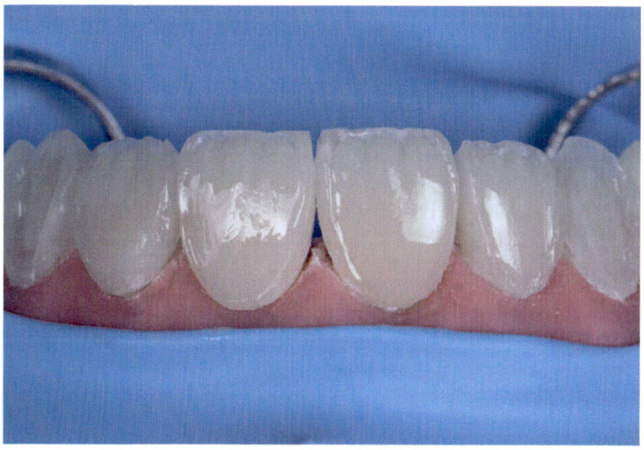

Figure 17 Single mass characterization technique.

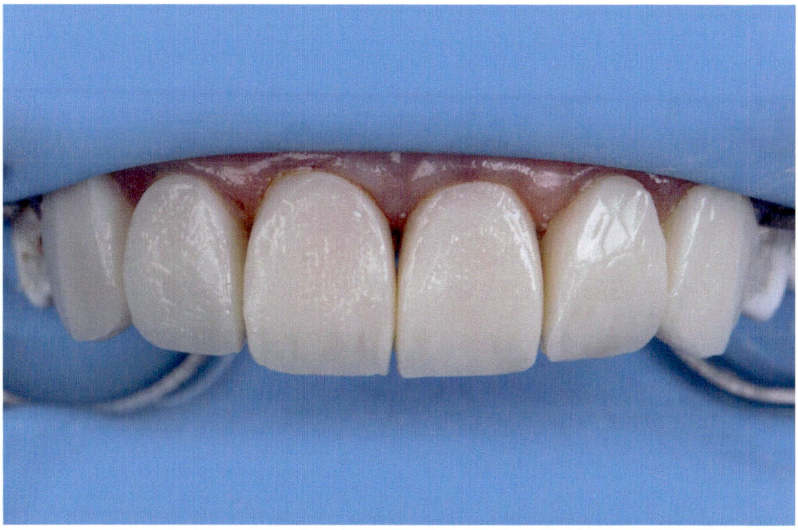

Figure 18 Smooth surface after final layering.

Simplified finishing and polishing steps will be divided into four steps (19):

1. Shape contouring by using a coarse disc at low speed.
2. Surface texture created by using Perio diamond bur.
3. Pre-polishing and surface smoothening by using twisted rubber (EVE Twist Diacomp, Germany).
4. Finally, polishing by using one-step Star Felt with diamond paste (Lucida).

A pencil is taken to draw the three facial planes following the labial curvature, the mesiodistal half curvature to follow the curve of the arch, the transitional mesial and distal lines, and finally the secondary and tertiary anatomies[20].
Starting at the cervical 45 degrees, move on all anterior teeth simultaneously.
Then mark the middle third for all the teeth at the same time.
Finally, mark the incisal third to ensure that all the teeth follow the three facial planes (20).

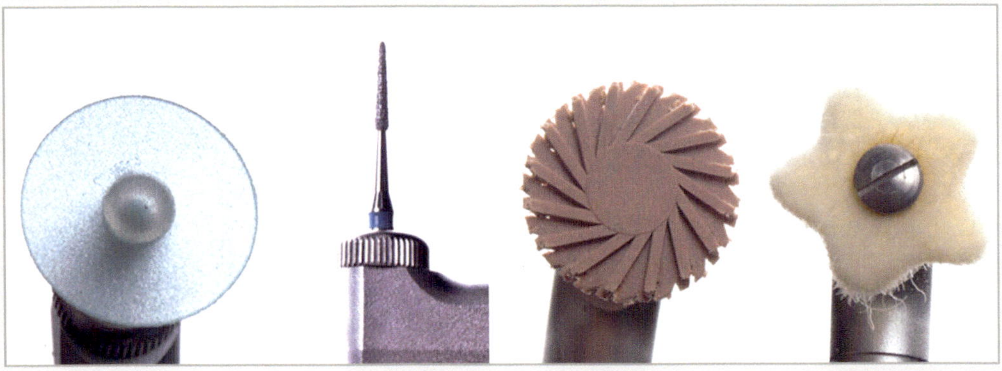

Figure 19 Photo of simplified finishing and polishing steps.

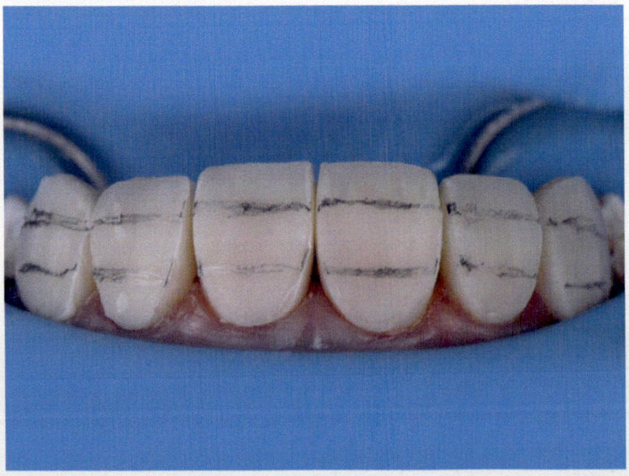

Figure 20 Finishing the three facial planes.

The labial surface should be divided into mesial and distal halves along the tooth-long axis. The mesial half of the two centrals at the same level and curvature should be finished together, then, the distal of centrals and the mesial of laterals and in the end, the distal of laterals and the mesial of canines.

After that, the disc is moved from cervical to incisal for the two mesial surfaces of the central incisors.

Then the distal of centrals and mesial of laterals and the same for the remaining teeth. (20a).

First, draw the transitional lines or light lines using a thin-tip pencil to control the lines in narrow areas, especially proximal ones (20b).

After drawing the transitional lines mesially and distally, use a caliper to measure the mesiodistal width, starting with a narrower diameter. It is easy to make wider look narrower, not the opposite (20c).

After measuring the diameter of the first and transferring it to the adjacent, draw the lines for the adjacent tooth (20d).

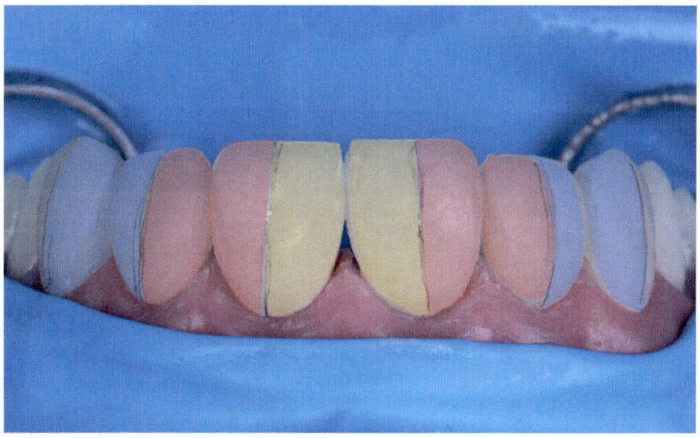

Figure 20a Mesiodistal half curvature finishing.

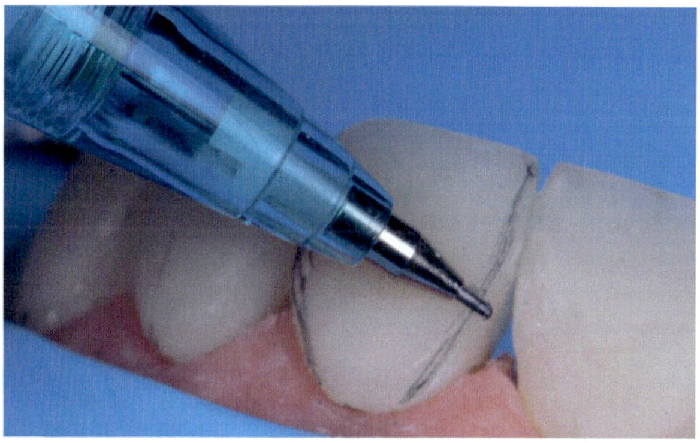

Figure 20b Photo of transitional lines.

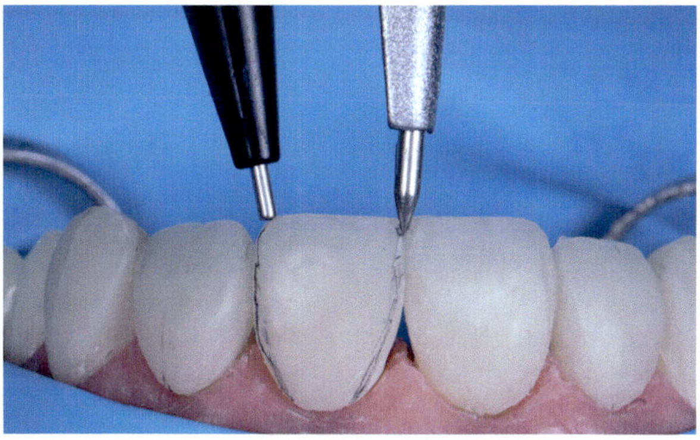

Figure 20c Measuring the width.

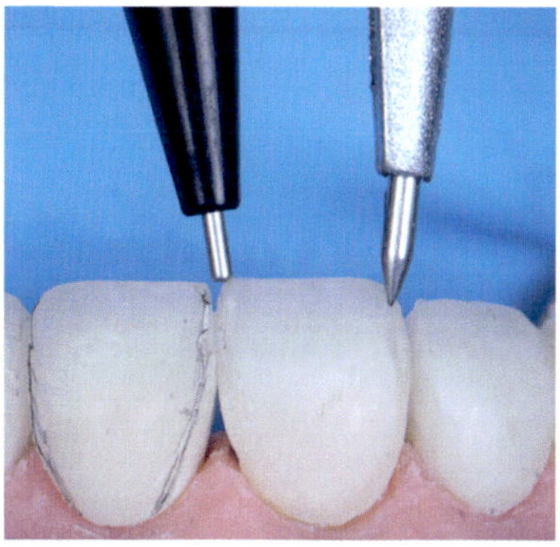

Figure 20d Transferring the width.

The area between the yellow zones is responsible for determining the width of the tooth and the light reflection area by making an illusion of a narrower or a wider tooth. If they are very close together, the yellow zones will give an illusion of a narrower tooth. Moreover, moving them away from each other, will provide an illusion of a wider tooth. This illusion will not appear until after the final surface gloss has been finished **(20e)**. The disc can be applied gently to the proximal surface because it is flexible and moved from inside the interproximal area to outside toward the lines to avoid opening the contact. This is done repetitively on the contralateral side until a symmetrical width is achieved **(20f)**.

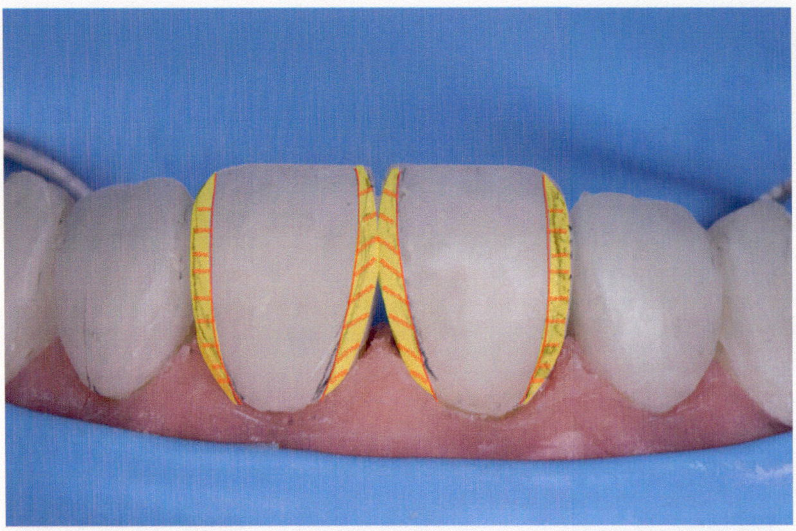

Figure 20e Light reflection area.

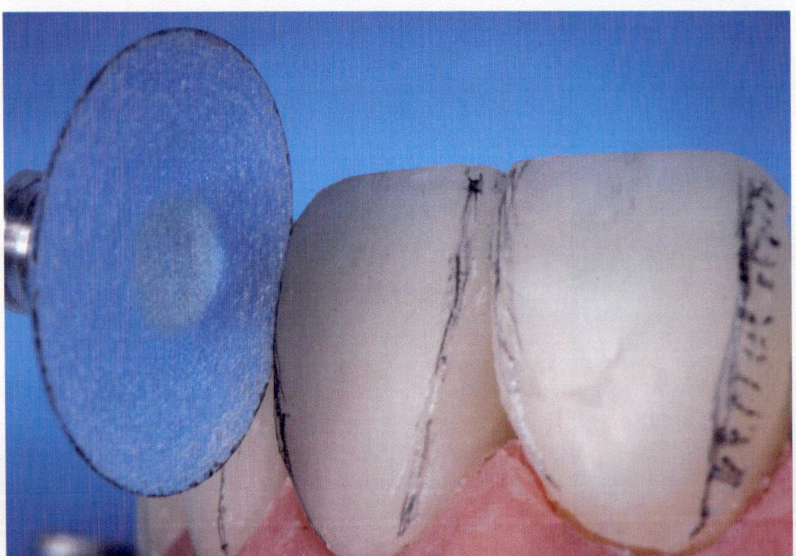

Figure 20f Using a disc from inside interproximal to outside.

The vertical macrotexture is usually more apparent with the V-shaped grooves. They are more open in the incisal and go narrower to the cervical.
Use the diamond Perio bur blue and red coded (Intensive, Switzerland) at low speed to make the secondary anatomy wider incisally and narrower cervically[20,24] (📷 21).
By using a twist rubber (EVE-twist polisher, Germany) that can be adapted easily to all surface details, labial and proximal, in a 45-degree arc from cervical to incisal with intermittent touch. When compared to a disc, the active end of the rubber is considered the end side, not the body.
After pre-polishing, the surface is very smooth, and the initial shine is evident on the surface (📷 22).

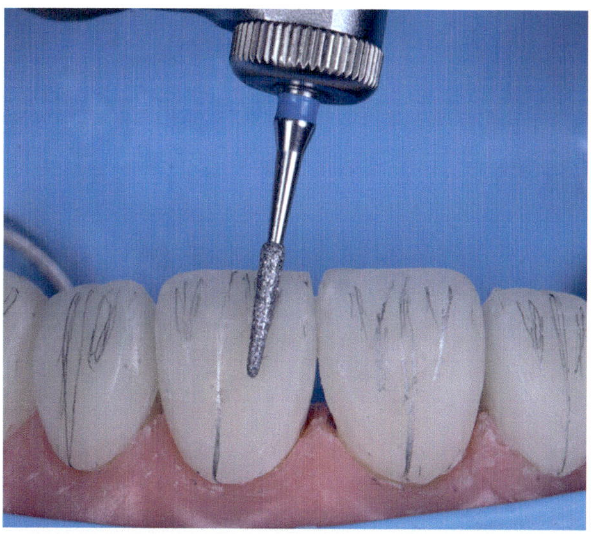

Figure 21 Using the diamond Perio bur to create surface texture.

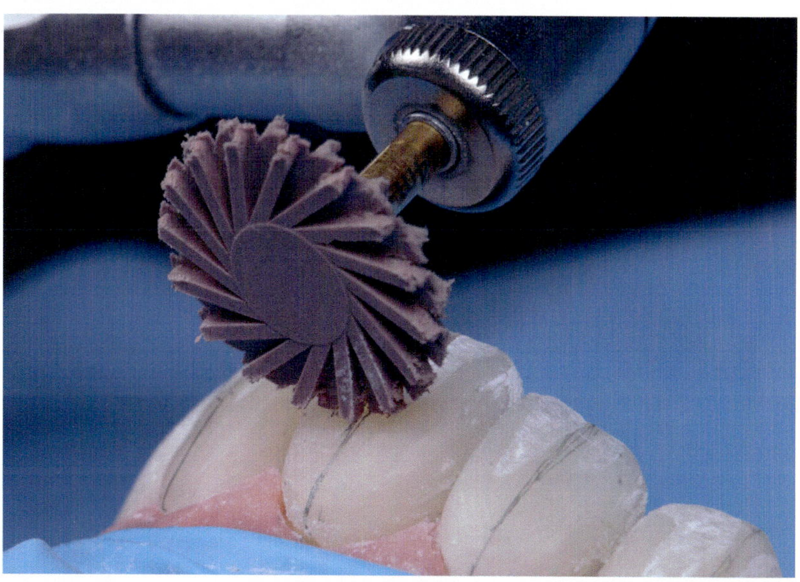

Figure 22 Twist rubber in action.

Lucida paste, and star shape felt for final polishing (Diashine, USA). Polishing is creating a very smooth and shiny surface by rubbing the surface or applying an abrasive material, leaving a clean surface with a significant specular reflection[14].

There are many polishing systems on the market. StyleItaliano has developed a new simple and fast method for the one-step universal polishing. It's called the Lucida composite gloss system.

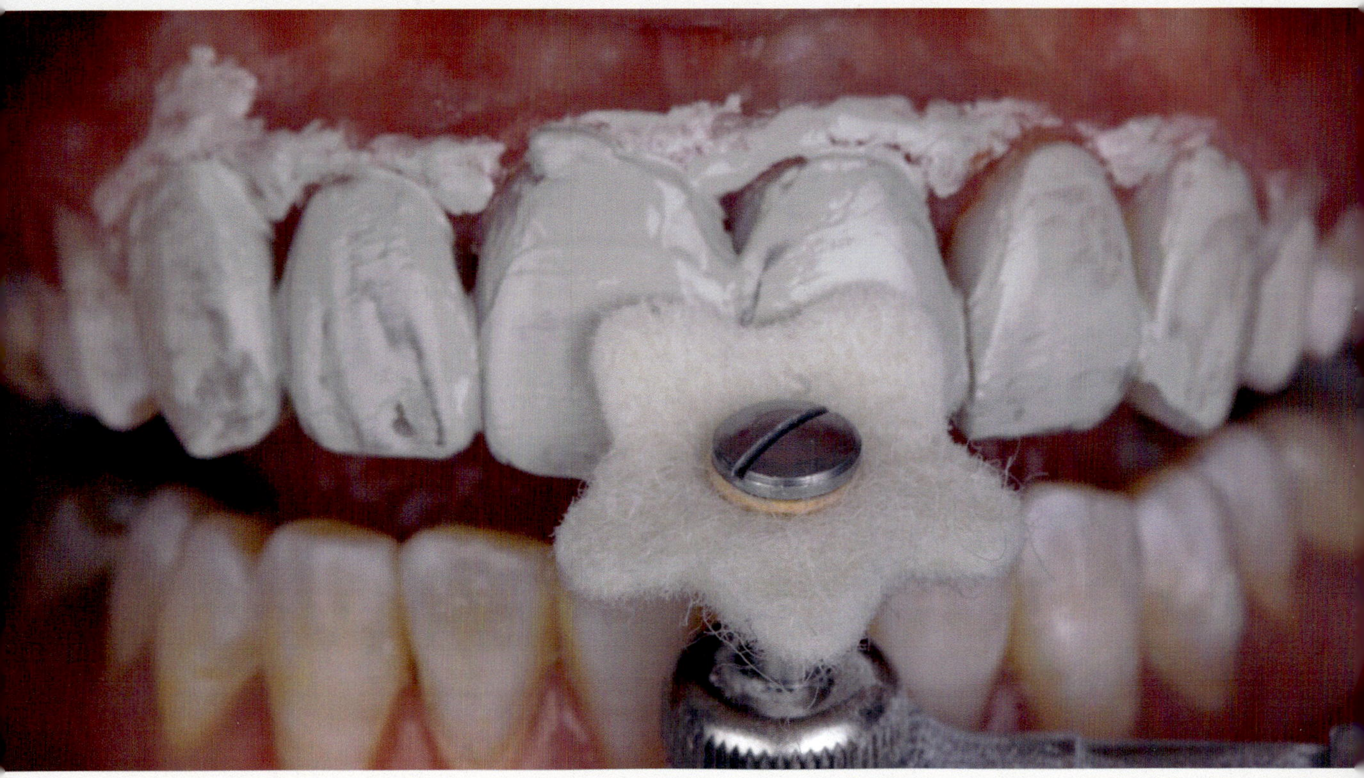

Figure 23 Final polishing.

Why use Lucida polishing?

- Autoclavable and reusable: the latch mandrel for the Lucida Star Felt is autoclavable and ready to be reused.
- Rounded angle shapes: thanks to Lucida Star rounded angles; it is now possible to reach narrow areas and get the desired intermittent touch[30].
- Variable thickness: Lucida Stars acquire a variable thickness depending on the pressure and speed applied. In addition, using the Lucida system saves time, and the combined solution with Lucida Paste and Lucida Star felt allows for single-step polishing of composite restorations (📷 23).

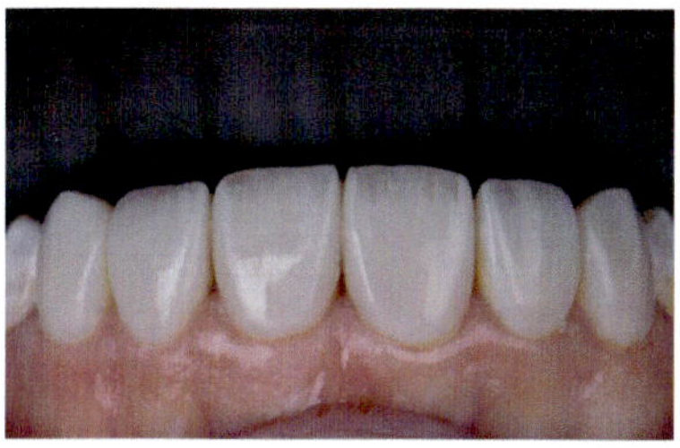

Figure 24 Final situation.

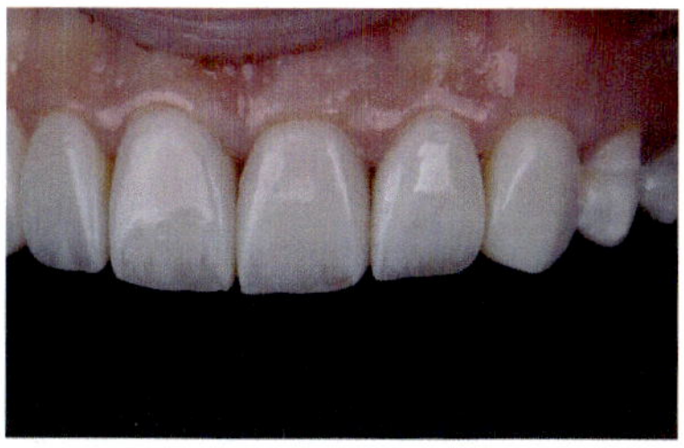

Figure 25 Side view-left.

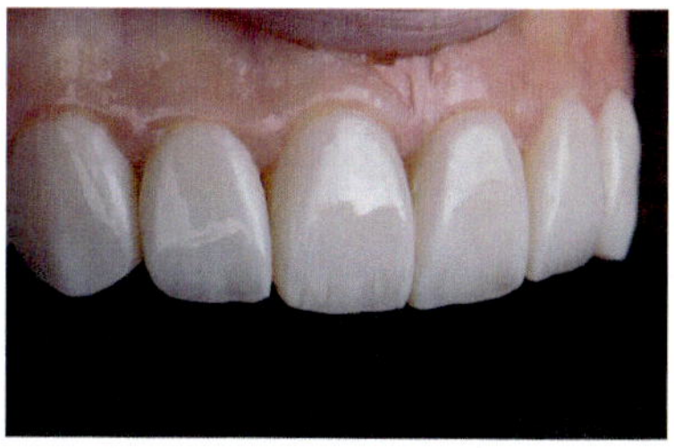

Figure 26 Side view-right.

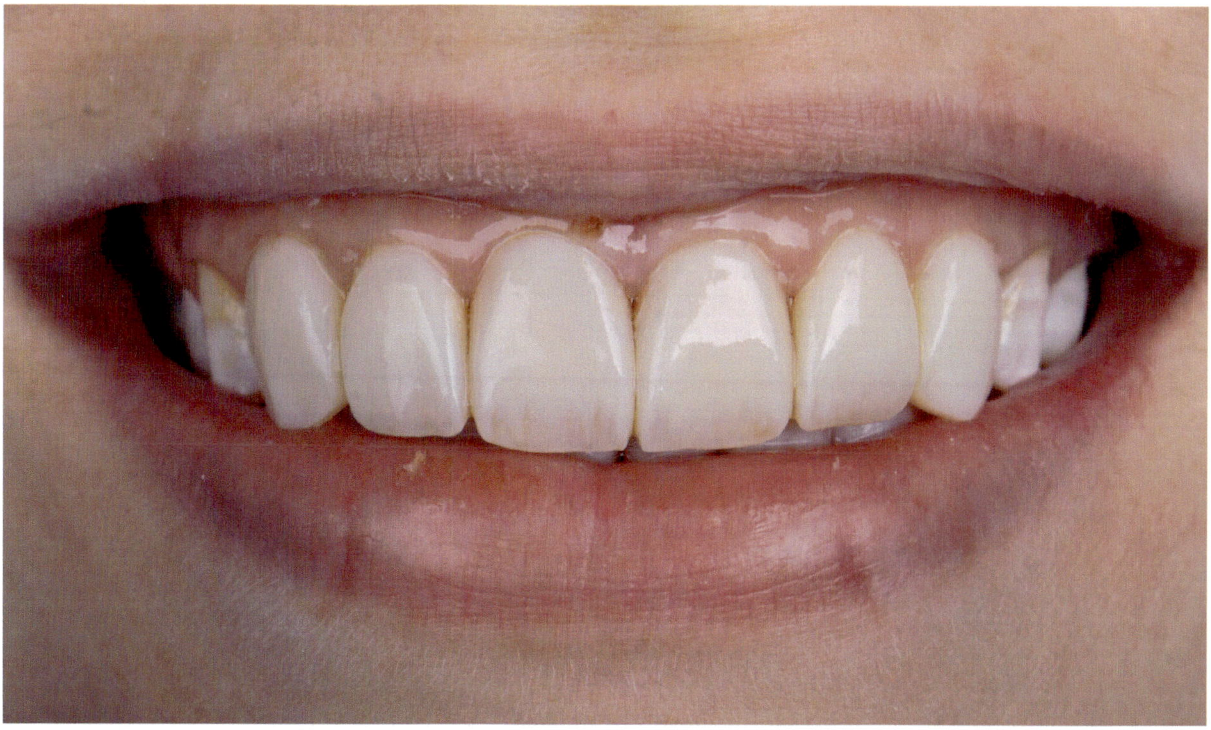

Figure 27 Full smile.

Dangerous areas to be considered

1. Midline

Any deviation in the midline will affect the symmetry and the final shape of the restorations (28).

2. Central dominance

The focus should be always on the central as any differences in the central incisors will be more readily noticeable than discrepancies in the lateral incisors or the canines[27] (29).

3. Mesial surface reflection

The transitional lines or light lines are one of the most important things that give the restoration a beautiful and pleasing effect if there are symmetrical reflections on both sides [2,14] (30).

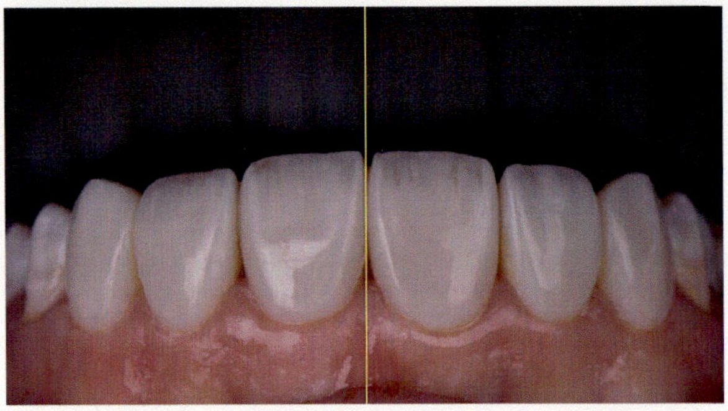

Figure 28 Midline.

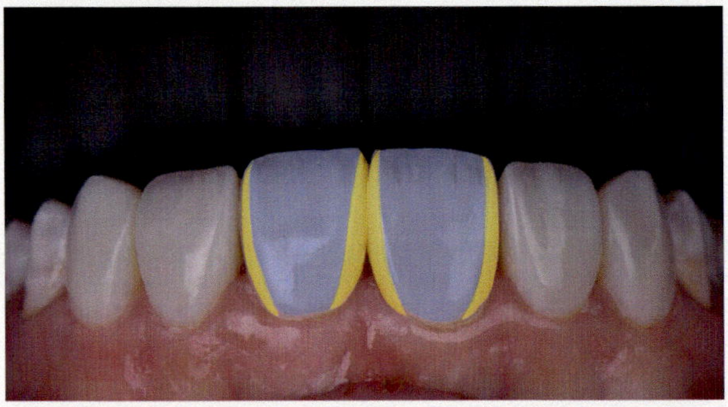

Figure 29 Central dominance.

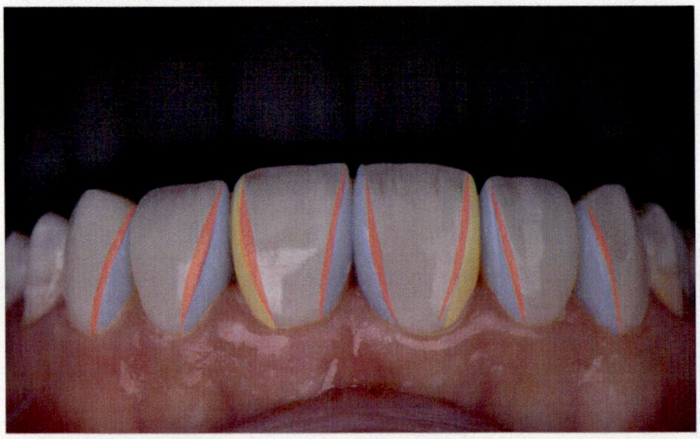

Figure 30 Mesial surfaces.

4. Contact area

Contact area, an aesthetic relationship has been suggested to exist between the anterior teeth, which is referred to as the "50-40-30 rule". This suggests that the ideal contact area between the two central incisors is 50% of the length of the central, between the maxillary central and lateral incisor it is 40% the length of the crown of the central incisor, and between the lateral incisor and the canine is 30% the length of the central incisor crown[2,13] (📷 31).

5. Incisal embrasures

The depth of the incisal embrasure between the next two teeth is usually a bit deeper, and it continues going a little deeper as the teeth move more toward the back teeth. This is a characteristic of natural teeth[2,15,26] (📷 32).

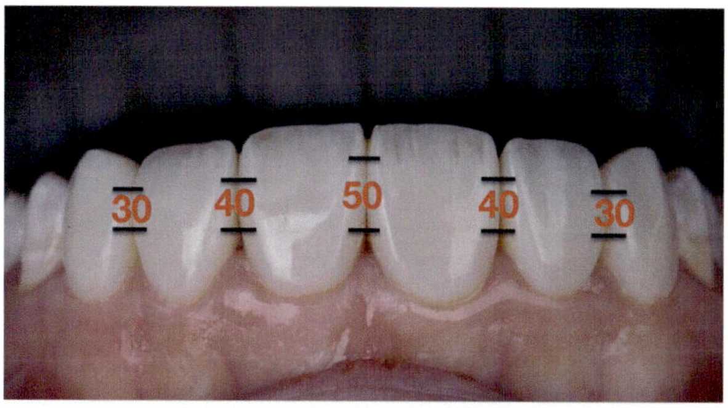

Figure 31 Contact area.

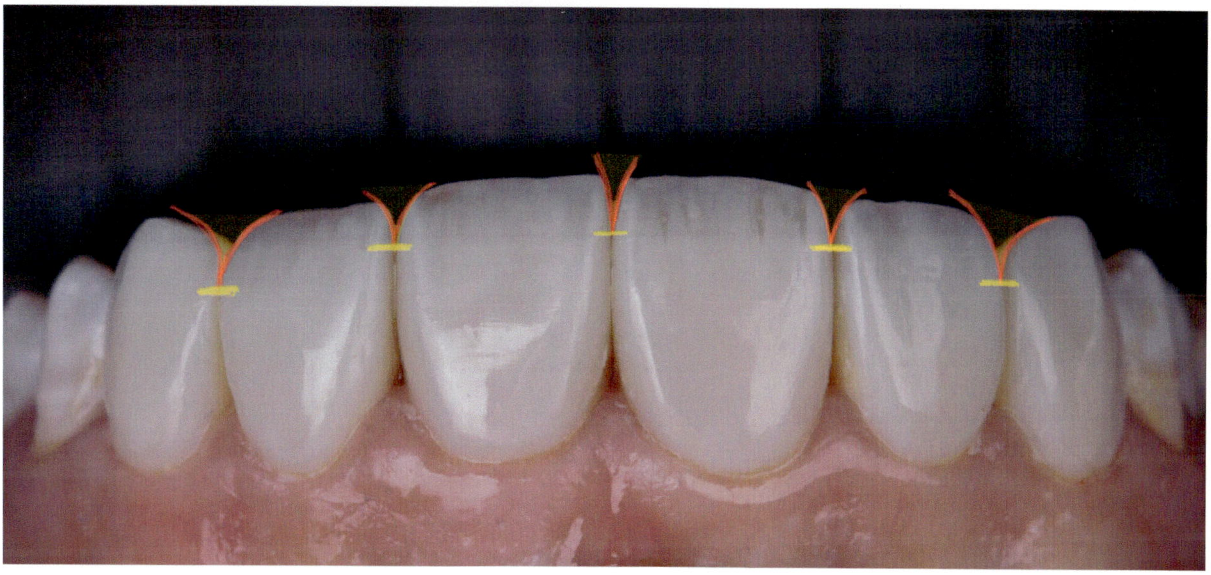

Figure 32 Incisal embrasures.

BIBLIOGRAPHY

1. Meyfarth S, da Silva CM, Antunes LS, Antunes LAA. Aesthetic-functional reconstruction of dental fracture and its impact on the psychosocial aspect. *Int J Burns Trauma.* 2021;11(4):328–336.
2. Magne P, Salem P, Magne M. Influence of symmetry and balance on visual perception of a white female smile. *J Prosthet Dent.* 2018;120(4):573-582.
3. Schmidt CJ, Tatum SA. Cosmetic dentistry. *Curr Opin Otolaryngol Head Neck Surg.* 2006;14(4):254-9.
4. Cardoso MV, de Almeida Neves A, Mine A, Coutinho E, Van Landuyt K, De Munck J, Van Meerbeek B. Current aspects on bonding effectiveness and stability in adhesive dentistry. *Aust Dent J.* 2011;56 Suppl 1:31-44
5. Perdigão J, Araujo E, Ramos RQ, Gomes G, Pizzolotto L. Adhesive dentistry: Current concepts and clinical considerations. *J Esthet Restor Dent.* 2021;33(1):51–68.
6. Demarco FF, Collares K, Correa MB, Cenci MS, Moraes RR, Opdam NJ. Should my composite restorations last forever? Why are they failing? *Braz Oral Res.* 2017;31(suppl 1):e56.
7. Araujo E, Perdigão J. Anterior Veneer Restorations–An Evidence-based Minimal-Intervention Perspective. *J Adhes Dent.* 2021;23(2):91–110.
8. Freeman R, Main JR, Burke FJ. Occupational stress and dentistry: theory and practice. Part I. Recognition. *Br Dent J.* 1995;178(6):214–7.
9. Kulkarni S, Dagli N, Duraiswamy P, Desai H, Vyas H, Baroudi K. Stress and professional burnout among newly graduated dentists. *J Int Soc Prev Community Dent.* 2016;6(6):535–541.
10. Mackenzie L, Parmar D, Shortall AC, Burke FJ. Direct anterior composites: a practical guide. *Dent Update.* 2013;40(4):297–9, 301–2, 305–8 passim.
11. Perdigão J. Current perspectives on dental adhesion: (1) Dentin adhesion-not there yet. *Jpn Dent Sci Rev.* 2020;56(1):190-207.
12. Wang Y, Li C, Yuan H, Wong MC, Zou J, Shi Z, Zhou X. Rubber dam isolation for restorative treatment in dental patients. *Cochrane Database Syst Rev.* 2016;9(9):CD009858.
13. Khan M, Kazmi SMR, Khan FR, Samejo I. Analysis of different characteristics of smile. *BDJ Open.* 2020;6:6.
14. Joiner A. Tooth colour: a review of the literature. *J Dent.* 2004;32 Suppl 1:3–12.
15. Eduarda Assad Duarte M, Martins Machado R, Fonseca Jardim da Motta A, Nelson Mucha J, Trindade Motta A. Morphological Simulation of Different Incisal Embrasures: Perception of Laypersons, Orthodontic Patients, General Dentists and Orthodontists. *J Esthet Restor Dent.* 2017;29(1):68–78.
16. Wang Q, Meng Q, Meng J. Minimally invasive esthetic management of dental fluorosis: a case report. *J Int Med Res.* 2020;48(10):300060520967538.
17. Romero MF, Babb CS, Delash J, Brackett WW. Minimally invasive esthetic improvement in a patient with dental fluorosis by using microabrasion and bleaching: A clinical report. *J Prosthet Dent.* 2018;120(3):323–326.
18. Ermis RB, De Munck J, Cardoso MV, Coutinho E, Van Landuyt KL, Poitevin A, Lambrechts P, Van Meerbeek B. Bonding to ground versus unground enamel in fluorosed teeth. *Dent Mater.* 2007;23(10):1250–5.
19. Hardan L, Bourgi R, Cuevas-Suárez CE, Lukomska-Szymanska M, Monjarás-Ávila AJ, Zarow M, Jakubowicz N, Jorquera G, Ashi T, Mancino D, Kharouf N, Haikel Y. Novel trends in dental color match using different shade selection methods: a systematic review and meta-analysis. *Materials.* 2022;15(2):468.

CONCLUSIONS

Once the dentists have mastered the SI simplified approach for direct veneering, smile makeovers and restorative work will result in drastically reduced chair time and overcome the daily challenges.

All cases can be done in a single visit without a wax-up step, thus decreasing the time and the budget for the patient.

The StyleItaliano simplified approach minimizes the number of instruments, materials, and steps during work.

This does not require a lot of skills because it is easy to master and not stressful.

By using the proper techniques, materials, and instruments, the simplified approach will make daily direct work more predictable and repeatable.

The simplest treatment option should always be considered, especially if it's the one meeting the patient's needs and wishes.

20. Manauat J, Salat A. Layers: An Atlas of Composite Resin Stratification. *Quintessence Pub.* 2013.

21. Hugo B. *Esthetics with Resin Composite: Basics and Techniques. Quintessence Pub.* 2009.

22. Devoto W, Pansecchi D. Composite restorations in the anterior region: clinical and aesthetic performances. *Pract Proced Aesthet Dent.* 2007;19(8):465–467.

23. LeSage B, Milner F, Wohlberg J. Achieving the epitome of composite art: creating natural tooth esthetics, texture and anatomy using appropriate preparation and layering techniques. *J Cosmet Dent.* 2008;24(3):132–141.

24. LeSage B. Finishing and polishing criteria for minimally invasive composite restorations. *Gen Dent. (Special cosmetic dentistry edition)* 2011;November/December:422–428.

25. Dabbagh s, Hardan I, Kassis C, Bourgi R, Devoto W, et al. Effect of intraoral humidity on dentin bond strength of two universal adhesives: an in vitro preliminary study. *Coatings, MDPI.* 2022;12(5)712.

26. Foulger TE, Tredwin CJ, Gill DS, Moles DR. The influence of varying maxillary incisal edge embrasure space and interproximal contact area dimensions on perceived smile aesthetics. *Br Dent J.* 2010;209(3):E4.

27. Alsulaimani FF, Batwa W. Incisors' proportions in smile esthetics. *J Orthod Sci.* 2013;2(3):109–12.

28. Korkut B. Smile makeover with direct composite veneers: A two-year follow-up report. *J Dent Res Dent Clin Dent Prospects.* 2018;12(2):146–151.

29. Pham TAV, Nguyen PA. Morphological features of smile attractiveness and related factors influence perception and gingival aesthetic parameters. *Int Dent J.* 2022;72(1):67–75.

30. Manauta J, Salat A, Devoto W, Putignano A. Layers 2, Direct Composites: The StyleItaliano Clinical Secrets. *Quintessence Pub.* 2020.